Boost Your Child's Immune System

What you need to know about allergies, vaccinations, antibiotics and diet, including over 160 recipes

Lucy Burney

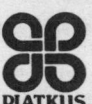

PIATKUS

First published in 2001 by
Judy Piatkus (Publishers) Limited
5 Windmill Street
London W1T 2JA

e-mail: info@piatkus.co.uk

The moral right of the author has been asserted

A catalogue record for this book is available from the British Library

ISBN 0 7499 2442 X

Text design and make up by Paul Saunders

This book has been printed on paper manufactured
with respect for the environment using wood from
managed sustainable resources

Data manipulation by Phoenix Photosetting, Chatham, Kent
Printed and bound in Great Britain by Mackays Ltd, Chatham, Kent

To Indy

CONTENTS

ACKNOWLEDGEMENTS

THIS BOOK HAS BEEN a true labour of love and there are a number of people whom I would like to thank for their part in making it happen. My thanks go to Laura Morris, my agent, and Rachel Winning, my editor, for their support and constructive advice; to Lynne McTaggart and Dotti Irving, who both gave their time to offer advice; to my sister Sarah and her nanny Michele, for testing endless recipes on family and friends; to my parents, for their years of support and encouragement; and finally to my Nige, who is as positive about the world as it is possible to be. For that and many other things, I am so very grateful.

Author's note

The material in this book is for information purposes only. It is not intended as an alternative to medical advice. If you suspect your child is suffering from a medical condition, you should always consult a doctor.

I have found myself referring to 'she' throughout the book. This is because I had my daughter, Indy, while I was writing it and have dedicated it to her. However, it is meant to refer to children of both sexes.

INTRODUCTION

HEALTHY CHILDREN HAVE strong immune systems. Strong immune systems are formed by the foods they eat. A healthy diet will not only help to keep them well when they're young, but also build up their resistance to disease and protect them in later life.

Over the last fifty years we have seen a dramatic decline in the quality of our children's diet. Recent research has shown that, even in the aftermath of the Second World War, children growing up in the fifties had a healthier diet than those of today. A study in December 1999 by the Medical Research Council revealed that nowadays children eat nearly twice as much sugar, have a lower fibre intake and consume fewer vitamins and minerals. The most recent National Diet and Nutrition survey published in June 2000 on four- to eighteen-year- olds showed that young people of this age group are on average eating less than half the recommended five portions of fruit and vegetables a day. One in five of those surveyed ate no fruit at all during the week of the survey. The most commonly consumed foods were white bread, savoury snacks, chips, biscuits, potatoes and chocolate confectionery. Fizzy soft drinks were the most popular beverage, with the younger children consuming on average 1.5 litres (2½ pints) a week.

With over 70 per cent of their diet consisting of sweets, chips and junk foods, we are raising a generation of undernourished 'junk food junkies'. Our children's diets are too high in saturated fat, sugar and salt, and this is not without its consequences. Feeding your children on this type of diet will suppress their immune systems and make them more susceptible to disease. The UK Office for National Statistics released a report on young people in June 2000 which showed one in five teenagers and young adults (aged between thirteen and twenty-four) reported a long-standing illness in 1998–9 compared to one in eight in 1975.

In the UK alone, approximately 4.5 million prescriptions for antibiotics were written for the under-sixteens in 1998. Half a million people in the UK are believed to contract food poisoning every year, many of these being children. One in four of the population is now affected by allergies and half of the sufferers are children. According to Cancer Research Campaign figures, cancer rates in the under-twenties rose by an alarming 27 per cent between 1971 and 1993. And these figures are similar throughout the Western world.

Obviously diet is not the sole culprit for the rise in ill health of our nation's children. Environmental pollution plays a significant part as our air becomes ever more congested with unwanted chemicals and other pollutants. Our genetic inheritance also plays an important part, as well as other more immediate factors. Our exposure to antibiotics from over-frequent prescriptions and the residues present in the food we eat have resulted in the birth of antibiotic-resistant 'superbugs' which pose a major health threat to the population as a whole. Additionally, some health professionals are singling out the continuing expansion of the mass immunisation programme for babies as yet another possible cause of immune suppression in the young.

This book is about making a difference. It is a positive step forward for a new generation of super-fit youngsters. Children do get ill; it is an important part of building their immunity.

What they do not need is an endless stream of prescriptions and over-the-counter drugs to suppress their symptoms and interfere with the body's natural ability to heal itself. What children do need is food that is going to strengthen their defences and make them better able to fight off bugs and infections – food that is fresh and full of immune-boosting nutrients. Whether you have a baby, a teenager or both, it is never too late to help improve your family's immunity. An immune-boosting diet is the key to their future health.

How to use this book

This book is designed for parents with children of all ages from birth to eighteen. Each age group has its own chapter which includes recipes that contain plenty of the nutrients that are especially important for that age group. The sections are broken down into:

- birth to six months
- six to nine months
- nine to twelve months
- one to four years
- five to twelve years
- thirteen to eighteen years

However, many of the recipes can be eaten by any of the age groups, adults included. For example, my five- and four-year-olds love Seafood Paella, even though I have put it in the teenage section. Experiment with the whole range of recipes to find your family's favourites.

As a working mother of three, I know the challenges involved in preparing hassle-free healthy food for children. This book has the answers. Whether it's five-minute meals you are looking for or menu ideas for hungry teenagers, the information is all within these pages.

I have also tried to make the recipes as user-friendly as possible. Formal measurements are used only where really necessary, and the use of 'handfuls', 'cups', 'tablespoons' and 'a piece of . . .' is liberal. Don't be alarmed if I don't mention the size of a vegetable required – it just means that the size will not affect the outcome of the recipe. It also makes for much easier shopping!

You will notice throughout the book that I have not separated the fish, poultry, meat, game, vegetarian or vegan recipes. This is to encourage you not to stick with familiar foods or recipes but to be more adventurous with your menu choices. The index, however, does group these recipes for you.

All the recipes can be easily halved or doubled to suit your family's requirements. The recipes in the baby chapters (Chapters 7, 8 and 9) serve one baby or are for batch cooking, and if this is the case the number of ice cube portions it will make is stated. But treat this only as a guide – amounts will vary according to the size of your ice cube trays, the size of your vegetables and the amount of extra liquid you may or may not add to suit your baby's particular preferences. The recipes in the one to four years chapter (Chapter 10) and the five to twelve years chapter (Chapter 11) are for two adults and two children unless stated otherwise in the recipe itself. They are generous in serving amounts, and will therefore feed two hungry adults and two children. The teenage recipes (thirteen to eighteen years, Chapter 12) will serve four adults. Each recipe is also coded to indicate whether it is wheat-free, dairy-free, gluten-free, vegetarian or vegan (see key below). This, I hope, will help you plan for all your family's different needs as they grow up.

Key to recipes

(**V**) = vegetarian   [df] = dairy-free

(**V**) = vegan   [gf] = gluten-free

[wf] = wheat-free   * = can be frozen

PART ONE

•

Your Child's Immune System

Understanding how your child's immune system works will enable you to keep her in optimum health. This section includes advice on dealing with allergies, antibiotics and vaccinations as well as how to boost your child's immunity.

Chapter 1

·

HOW IT WORKS

Every minute of every day, your child is exposed to germs that exist in her environment. Right from birth she adopts strategies to deal with them. Collectively, this is called her immune system.

This amazing piece of engineering is a complex maze of interconnecting systems, organs and cells. The immune system is often described as an army, as there are so many different types of forces which work together to protect your child's body from disease by attacking unwanted intruders such as viruses, bacteria, fungi and cancer cells. A lack of certain vitamins and minerals, or too much of the wrong kind of nutrients, causes the immune system to function much less effectively.

This chapter tells you about some of the body systems that make up the immune system. It uses a number of terms that may be unfamiliar, but don't be put off. They will be encountered frequently in later chapters when I describe what various nutrients do to improve your child's health via their immune system. There is also a Glossary at the back which defines many of the words repeatedly used throughout this book.

To prevent germs from entering your child's body, she has a plethora of physical attributes that form her first line of defence:

- The skin is a very effective barrier against bacteria. It contains large quantities of substances called unsaturated fatty acids, which are known to kill bacteria. Sweat also contains salt, another protective element.

- Tiny nose hairs and the hairs that line the respiratory tract sweep away inhaled intruders.

- Hydrochloric acid in the stomach kills off germs that are swallowed.

- Friendly bacteria in the gut prevent unwanted visitors from taking over.

- The flushing action of urine prevents urinary infections.

- Tears contain large quantities of lysozyme, a substance that can destroy bacteria.

If the intruders do get through this first line of defence, the immune army swings into action to form the second line of defence, at cell level.

The cells of the immune system

White blood cells

The main defenders of your child's immune system are the white blood cells. There are three main types:

- lymphocytes
- monocytes and macrophages
- granulocytes

Lymphocytes

The lymphocytes are the generals. Their job is to travel around the bloodstream and the lymphatic system, recognise any foreign invader, whether bacteria, virus or other infecting agent, and mount an organised attack against it. There are two main types of lymphocytes:

- T-lymphocytes
- B-lymphocytes

Both these types of cells develop from stem cells in the liver and bone marrow when your child is still in the womb. T-lymphocytes are so-called because they mature and/or are instructed in their duties in the thymus gland. The T-lymphocytes themselves are of three kinds:

- T-helpers
- T-suppressors
- NK (natural killer cells)

The T-helpers help to activate the B-lymphocytes to produce antibodies, whilst T-suppressors turn off the reactions once the invader has been destroyed and the battle won. Natural killer cells can produce toxins that will obliterate any invading organism.

Monocytes and macrophages

These two types of white blood cell finish off the battle by engulfing and digesting the invader by causing inflammation and alerting the other troops to their presence.

Granulocytes

The third type of white blood cell provides further back-up in the war against invaders.

Red blood cells

The main responsibility of these cells is to carry oxygen around the body. But they also have suction pads which can grab invaders and deliver them to a white blood cell for extermination.

The parts of the body that make up the immune system

The *lymphatic system* (see the diagram at the end of this chapter) is a pivotal part of your child's immune system. It consists of an internal network of vessels throughout the body that contains a clear liquid called lymph, which carries certain defence cells around the body. Unlike blood, which is pumped round the body by the heart, lymph relies on exercise and muscular activity in order to circulate.

The *lymph nodes* are storage sites for cells and are the field on which many an immunological battle is fought. These nodes are the 'swollen glands' often present during an infection.

The *tonsils, adenoids, appendix* and areas called *Peyer's patches* along the small intestine are other important lymphoid tissue.

The *thymus gland, bone marrow* and *spleen* are all sites where immune cells mature. In addition the thymus gland, just behind the breastbone, is responsible for programming all new cells with the body's own code. This ensures that, in the future, the body will not attack any cell with the 'me' marking. If this programming is not done properly it can result in autoimmune diseases such as rheumatoid arthritis and diabetes in later life.

The *liver,* too, is very important, because it helps to detoxify many substances in the body that could be taxing to your child's immune system.

Antibodies

The other really important troops in the immune army are the antibodies. At around six months, your baby will start to produce her own antibodies rather than continuing to rely on

---

Exercise and your child's immune system

According to the National Diet and Nutrition Survey, published in June 2000, 40 per cent of boys and 60 per cent of girls between six and fifteen years of age spend less than one hour a day on exercise. This statistic gets even worse in the fifteen-to-eighteen age bracket. Computer games and television are partly to blame. A staggering 24 per cent of under-fours have a television set in their bedrooms. As a result, obesity in this age group is on the increase.

Your child's immune system relies on exercise in order to function properly. Without exercise the lymph, whose job is to transport some of the immune army around the body, cannot move. So making sure your children get plenty of exercise will actively improve their resistance, whereas lack of exercise will increase their risk of frequent infections as the lymphatic system becomes sluggish and clogged up.

---

yours for protection. There are five types of antibodies, also known as immunoglobulins (Ig):

- **IgG antibodies** make up 75 per cent of the antibodies in the entire body. They protect against bacteria and viruses by neutralising toxins and preventing viruses from entering body cells. These are the antibodies that are passed on to your baby through the placenta.

- **IgA antibodies** are the major type found in breast milk, saliva, tears and respiratory and intestinal secretions. They prevent localised infection from spreading through the body.

- **IgM antibodies** are the first to mount an attack when exposed to a foreign invader.

- **IgE antibodies** are involved in allergic reactions.

- **IgD antibodies** undoubtedly have a particular function, but scientists have not yet discovered what it is.

Other important immune system components found in the blood:

- **Interferon:** an antiviral agent which protects uninfected cells from viral infection.

- **Complement:** proteins in the blood which come together when stimulated to destroy unwanted bacteria. Also triggers inflammation.

- **Transferrin:** an iron-binding protein which prevents bacterial multiplication. Bacteria are dependent on iron to multiply and they have to compete with transferrin. Low levels of transferrin increase susceptibility to infection, since the iron then becomes accessible to the invading micro-organism.

Does your child's immune system need boosting?

As with all body systems, balance is the key. A number of important nutrients are needed to enhance immune health. Without these nutrients your child's immune system can be suppressed and deficiency symptoms may occur. Frequent use of antibiotics and over-the-counter medicines can also be immune suppressive. Look at the chart on pages 8 and 9, if your child regularly suffers from any of the symptoms listed, she will benefit from following the immune-boosting diet.

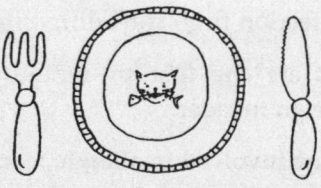

Dietry guide for boosting your child's immune system

Symptom	Indicates	Eat More
Frequent colds and infections	Possible antioxidant deficiency (lacking vitamins A, C and E, zinc and selenium)	Citrus fruit, berries, kiwi fruit, peppers, tomatoes, nuts and seeds, seafood
Slow wound healing and exhaustion after light exercise	Possible vitamin E deficiency	Avocados, nuts and seeds, unrefined oils, wheatgerm, oatmeal
Dry skin or eczema	Vitamin B12, B2, biotin and essential fatty acids (EFA) deficiencies	Seafood, wholegrains, poultry, game, nuts and seeds and their oils
Asthma	Possible magnesium and vitamin B6, B12 and C deficiency	Green leafy vegetables, nuts and seeds, wholegrains, egg yolks
Loss of appetite, white marks on nails, poor growth	Possible zinc deficiency	Shellfish, seeds, poultry and game
Pale skin, nausea, fatigue	Possible iron deficiency	Red meat, organic liver, green leafy vegetables, dried fruit, wholegrains
Mouth ulcers, pimples on back of arms, recurrent colds and infections, dull hair	Lack of vitamin A (beta-carotene)	Chicken liver, lamb's liver, green leafy vegetables, carrots, tomatoes, squashes, mangoes, peaches, apricots, sweet potatoes, papaya
Poor sleeping habits fatigue, grinding teeth, twitches, pins and needles, hyperactivity	Magnesium and/or calcium deficiency	Milk, yoghurt, nuts and seeds, green leafy vegetables, sardines, tinned salmon with bones, tofu, soya products

Eat Less	Recipes
Sugar and refined carbohydrates (white bread, cakes, biscuits, white pasta, white rice)	Bouillabaise (page 214); Berry Booster Yoghurt Lollies (page 152)
Fried foods, cakes, crisps, pastries	Pumpkin Seed Porridge (page 198); Yoghurt Mountain (page 153); Flapjacks (page 184); Roasted Nut and Vegetable Couscous (page 172)
Saturated fats, sugar, refined foods	Essential Fatty Acid Tonic (page 247); Muesli Bars (page 136); Venison Shepherd's Pie (page 151); Chicken Risotto (page 174)
Phytates, salt, sugar, Oxalates, saturated fat	Liquid Energy Breakfast (page 196); Red Lentil and Spinach Lasagne (page 146); Salmon Stir-fry (page 175)
Sugar, iron supplements,	Seafood Paella (page 212); Nut and Seed Bread (page 229); Turkey Burgers (page 145); Immune-boosting Venison excess phytates (page 228)
Fizzy drinks (phosphates), excess phytates, zinc supplements	Protein-packed Porridge (page 137); Trace Element Tonic (page 246); Baked Duck with Honey and Mustard Marinade (page 226)
Sugar	Juice Boost (page 244); Butternut Squash Risotto ; (page 141) Chicken Liver Medley (page 126); Quick and Easy Chicken Liver Pâté (page 200)
	Almond Tofu Stir-fry (page 176); Panna (page 211); Quick Nut Burgers (page 206); Pumpkin Seed Porridge (page 198); Fruitful (page 197)

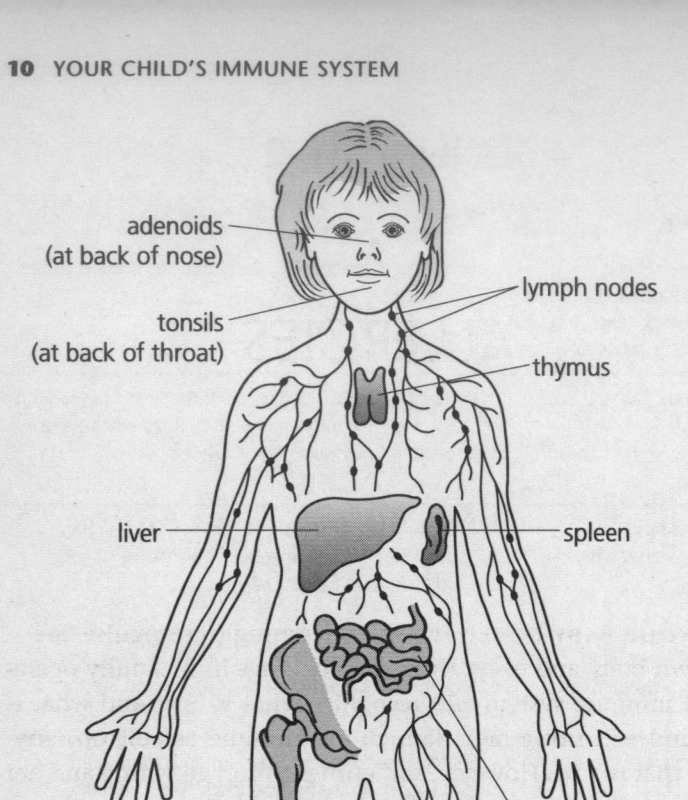

adenoids
(at back of nose)

lymph nodes

tonsils
(at back of throat)

thymus

liver

spleen

Peyers patches
in intestines

bone marrow

lymphatic
vessels

The lymphatic system

Chapter 2

·

ALLERGIES

As your baby develops she is learning to recognise 'me' – her own body and every thing that belongs in it. A fully operational immune system will recognise what is 'me' and what is not, and will not attack (launch an immune assault on) anything that is 'me'. However, sometimes things go wrong and her immune system can respond to harmless or even useful things as though they were enemies. When the immune system attacks something that enters her body, such as a particular food or an environmental particle such as pollen, that is called an allergy. When it attacks her body itself, as in the case of rheumatoid arthritis or juvenile diabetes, that is called an autoimmune disease.

In May 2000, according to the UK Eczema Society, as many as one in five children now suffer from eczema. The latest asthma audit (1999/2000) by the National Asthma Campaign revealed that one in seven children in the UK now has asthma. This same audit estimated that over one third of children between two and fifteen take more than a week off school per year due to asthma – 8 per cent miss more than one month.

Quite why allergies have escalated in this alarming way remains a mystery. It is possible that the increased chemical burden on our immune system is partly responsible, or that genetically we are acquiring weakened immunity through the generations. Some blame the 'hygiene hypothesis' (see page 23). However, without doubt environmental pollution plays its part. We are now exposed to over 7,000 chemicals on a daily basis, from the food we eat and the air that we breathe, which must place a heavy burden on adult bodies, let alone those of our children's. Poor diet, lacking in the essential nutrients required for a strong immune system, is another contributing factor. Early exposure to foods is also a possible cause: a baby's intestines are immature and therefore porous, allowing particles to pass through the intestinal wall into the bloodstream where the immune system identifies an unwanted intruder and launches an assault. This sets up an allergic reaction.

Some allergies run in the family, a condition called atopy. If you yourself have, for example, asthma, eczema, hay fever or migraine, then your child runs a 40 per cent risk of developing one of these conditions – although it may not necessarily be the same one as you. If both you and your partner have allergies, the risk rises to 60 per cent.

Allergies and similar reactions at a glance

- Allergies are caused by the immune system attacking something from outside the body, e.g. a particular food.
- Autoimmune disease is the result of the immune system attacking the body itself.
- Inherited allergies are called atopy.
- Type I allergy (IgE) is a classic food allergy evoking an immediate response.
- Type II allergy (IgG) is food intolerance/sensitivity, evoking a delayed response.

Food allergy and intolerance

Food allergies affect one in twenty children under the age of four. Fortunately, most grow out of them and recent figures suggest that only 2 per cent of the adult population suffer from classic food allergies. It is important to distinguish the different types of allergy, as this is a grey area which can be confusing. A classic food allergy causes an immediate immune response and is called a Type I allergy (IgE) (see page 6). The first signs of an allergic response to a food are swelling lips and an itchy mouth. This may be followed by nausea, abdominal pain, diarrhoea and/or rashes. These and other symptoms are listed in the box overleaf. Occasionally asthma symptoms can occur in a child who is already asthmatic. If she has severe breathing problems, this is called an anaphylactic shock and requires immediate medical attention. In 90 per cent of cases, a food allergy is caused by one of the following foods:

- milk
- eggs
- soya
- wheat
- peanuts
- tree nuts (e.g. hazelnuts, pecans)
- sesame
- fish
- shellfish

Nut and fish allergies are unlikely to be grown out of. The sufferer will have to carry with them an antidote injection of adrenalin in case they unknowingly eat some of the food to which they are allergic. When weaning your baby, take care when introducing these foods and notice any adverse reaction. Anaphylactic shock is rare and will only occur on your child's second exposure to a food to which they are allergic.

A food intolerance or food sensitivity involves a different reaction altogether. It is often called a Type II allergy (IgG) and does not necessarily involve any immune response at all. A delayed response to a food, it can be difficult to isolate and is most frequently associated with foods eaten on a daily basis, such as bread and milk. Rotating foods (see page 13) and giving your children a wide variety of different ones will help to prevent food intolerances developing.

Quick check list of symptoms of an allergic reaction

- Swelling of lips, eyes, tongue
- Itching mouth
- Vomiting
- Diarrhoea
- Rashes
- Flushing
- Difficulty in breathing
- Abdominal pain

Quick check list of symptoms commonly associated with food intolerance or sensitivity

- Colic in babies
- Vomiting
- Persistent diarrhoea
- Poor appetite
- Recurrent ear infections
- Asthma
- Stomach aches
- Rash around the mouth
- Runny or congested cold
- Glue ear
- Eczema
- Urticaria (hives or nettle rash)
- Headaches
- Migraines
- Hyperactivity
- Aching muscles and joints
- Infantile insomnia
- Bedwetting

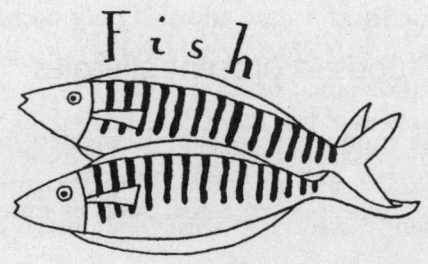

Preventing allergies

The good news is that, even if your child has an inherited predisposition for allergies, the right dietary approach can delay their onset and greatly reduce their severity. Here are some guidelines for preventing allergies.

Eight-point plan for preventing allergies

1. Breast-feed for six months exclusively

2. Include plenty of essential fatty acids (see page 47) in your diet whilst breastfeeding

3. Avoid weaning your baby on to solids until she is six months old

4. Follow the chart at the beginning of each recipe section (see pages 87, 113 and 135) for introducing foods to babies (asterisked items are potential allergy causers)

5. Keep a food diary to detect any adverse reactions to foods

6. Introduce foods slowly

7. Rotate foods, so that you do not rely on too few foods in your child's staple diet

8. Avoid processed foods full of additives, artificial colouring matter and heat-damaged oils (see page 56).

Rotating foods to prevent allergies

1. From the moment your baby is weaned, be aware of food you regularly give her. For breakfast, rather than always offering a wheat-based cereal such as muesli, Weetabix or

Shredded Wheat, on some days choose one of the oat-based recipes in this book, or use rye bread or Ryvita.

2. Once your child is drinking milk, alternate the different kinds – soya milk, rice milk, cow's milk and goat's milk. For example, I sometimes now cook with organic semi-skimmed milk, and my two boys tend to drink soya or rice milk.

3. Structure the day's meals so that you are not repeating the same food in different forms. For example, muesli and toast with milk for breakfast, followed by a sandwich and yoghurt at lunch and pasta for tea is a very typical day's menu for toddlers. But it is over-reliant on wheat and dairy products. A better combination would be porridge for breakfast, a sandwich and fruit for lunch, and rice pasta and vegetable sauce, followed by a yoghurt, for tea. These simple changes introduce far more variety into your children's diet and will help to prevent intolerances occurring.

4. Look at the lists of wheat- and dairy-free foods on page 22 to help you plan your week's meals. The menu plans at the end of each recipe section are good examples of rotating foods and food groups. As you can see, where possible wheat is not included more than once a day.

Treating food allergies

If you have an older child who you suspect has a food allergy or intolerance, don't despair – there are some simple steps that you can take to discover the culprit and relieve the symptoms. I often tell parents to look at their child's face for clues:

● Does your child have dark shadows under her eyes (allergic shiners)?

● Are there creases in her lower lids?

● Is her nose always running whether she has a cold or not?

● Does she often get red ears?

These are all facial symptoms of food allergy. The most common is the dark shadows under the eyes, which more often than not indicates a problem with wheat.

Ten-point plan for treating allergic children

1. Support your child's immune system by providing her with an organic, wholefood diet, rich in fruit and vegetables, grains, pulses and beans, unrefined oils and oily fish (from unpolluted waters: see Resources).

2. Make sure your child's diet is rich in essential fatty acids, found in nuts and seeds and their oils as well as oily fish. These fats convert into anti-inflammatory prostaglandins, which can help to control inflammatory responses. Children with atopic eczema appear to be lacking an enzyme needed for this conversion, but evening primrose oil rubbed on their skin or taken orally seems to work very well to reduce the inflammation. For a complete explanation of essential fatty acids, see page 47.

3. Make sure you include plenty of anti-allergy nutrients in your child's diet, including vitamin C. Calcium ascorbate or magnesium ascorbate are the best types of vitamin C for your child to take and they are available in powder form. A mineral ascorbate is a combination of vitamin C bound with a mineral and is less acidic than the most common form of vitamin C, ascorbic acid. Other important nutrients include bioflavonoids (especially quercetin, see page 48), zinc, calcium, magnesium and beta-carotene (see page 41).

4. If you suspect a particular food is causing a problem, the simplest answer is to remove it from your child's diet for a month. Paradoxically, this food could be the food they crave the most. This is because initially they feel great after eating the allergy-causing food, as natural morphine-like substances are released into the bloodstream to give your child a sort of 'high'. These substances, called exorphins, mimic the activity of our endorphins which are our natural pain-killers. Endorphins are released in the body in response to pain, strenuous exercise or stressful events and make us feel better. Ask your child if there is one food that they could not give up and you may be surprised by the answer! When you cut out the likely culprit food from your child's diet, read the labels of manufactured products carefully to avoid this food or any derivatives. Make sure you replace the food(s) on trial with suitable alternatives so that your child's diet remains high in nutritional value.

Here are some examples of hidden ingredients to help you decipher food labels in the supermarket:

Hidden sugar
- sucrose
- glucose
- lactose
- maltose
- fructose
- glucose syrup
- invert syrup
- hydrolysed starch
- treacle
- honey
- maple syrup

Disguised wheat
- semolina
- couscous
- spelt
- kamut
- flour
- cereal protein
- cereal starch
- cereal binder
- cereal filler

Hidden milk
- whey
- casein/caseinate
- lactalbumin
- lactose

Hidden soya

Around 6o per cent of the processed food we eat contains soya in one form or another:

- vegetable protein
- hydrolysed vegetable protein
- protein isolate
- textured vegetable protein
- lecithin
- vegetable oil
- vegetable fat
- hydrogenated vegetable oil

5. Keep a close eye on your child during the elimination period and see if anything changes: does she feel better, has her runny nose dried up, is she sleeping better, has she got more energy and so on. After the month is up reintroduce the food in its purest form. If your child was avoiding wheat, give her a bowl of plain pasta. If she was avoiding dairy products, give her a glass of milk. Take her pulse over a sixty-second period before she has the food and test it again ten minutes afterwards. If you can keep her quiet it is a good idea to take her pulse once again thirty minutes later, but this is not always practicable with young children. If her pulse goes up by more than ten points she may be reacting to that particular food and you should continue to avoid giving it to her for another month. It is interesting that after a period of avoidance (up to six months) the immune system often 'forgets' its reaction to the food, which can then be reintroduced.

Taking your child's pulse

Choose a time when your child is distracted; an ideal time could be while they watch a video. This is especially important for young children, because if they are jumping up and down or keep moving around, their pulse rate will inevitably rise!

Finding your child's pulse is really easy. You can either find it in their wrist or on their neck. On the wrist it is in the dip between the tendon and the bone on the inside of the wrist. On your child's neck the pulse can be found beneath the chin between the voice box and the ear. It is very strong in this area and some parents may find it easier to locate. Always use your fingers to locate and take the pulse and not your thumb as it carries your pulse which you may feel instead.

Remember to take your child's pulse and write it down:

1. before they eat the suspected food
2. straight after they have finished eating the food
3. ten minutes later.

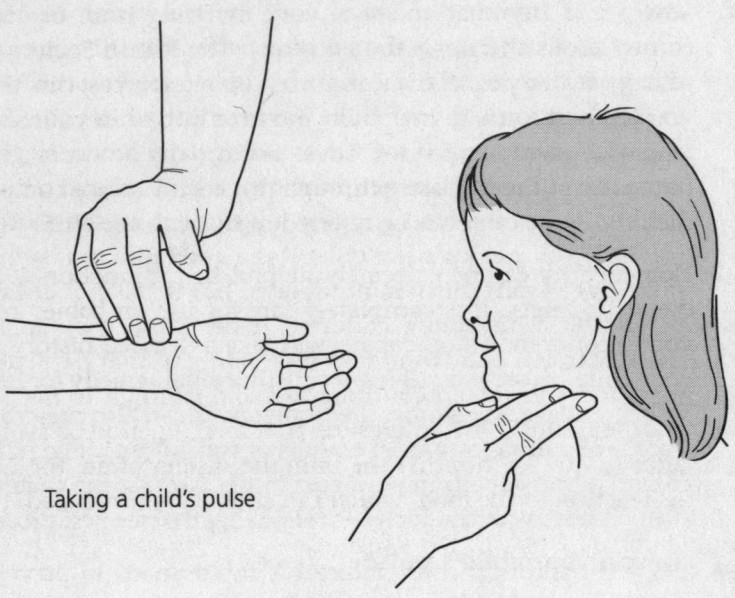

Taking a child's pulse

6. If you have no idea which foods are causing a problem, start with those that are the most likely:

- wheat
- dairy products
- eggs
- soya
- nuts
- corn
- citrus fruit

Yeast and sugar can also cause problems for some children, especially those who have been exposed to a lot of antibiotics. You can either put your child on an elimination diet or get some allergy tests done. Conventional allergy tests which your doctor can arrange are really only suitable for classic allergies and will not pick up food intolerances. An elimination diet should be a short-term event conducted under the guidance of a health professional to make sure that your child receives enough of the right kinds of nutrients despite the restrictions. The British Allergy Foundation offers general advice and information for anyone suffering from or concerned about allergies (see Resources). The British Society of Allergy and Environmental Medicine (see Resources) can give you the name of a nutritionally oriented doctor in your area who specialises in allergies. These doctors can be expensive, but many of them operate through private insurance companies and some can even be referred to through the NHS.

7. Homeopathy can be extremely helpful in conjunction with dietary changes. It is completely safe for use on babies and young children. A homeopath will take a detailed history of your child before prescribing a constitutional remedy for her. To help relieve symptoms, the homeopath can also prescribe remedies in drop form or as crystals or small dissolvable pills. To find a homeopath in your area either contact the Faculty of Homeopathy or the Society of Homeopaths (see Resources).

8. Once the intolerance is eradicated, rotate foods to prevent further intolerances occurring.

9. Give your children a daily multivitamin and mineral to ensure they are receiving adequate nutrients to strengthen and protect their immune system. When preparing food use ingredients such as garlic, ginger, cloves and green herbs for their immune-protecting properties.

10. Take your child for a nutritional MOT every couple of years to check you are on the right track (see Resources for nutritionally oriented doctors and other nutrition practitioners).

Coping with food exclusion

These lists contain alternatives to common foods such as wheat and dairy products, which you may be excluding from your child's diet for a while. All the recipes in this book are coded so that you can see at a glance which are dairy-free, wheat-free or gluten-free, as well as which are vegetarian or vegan.

Wheat-free foods	
Grains	Brown rice, millet, corn, barley, quinoa, oats, rye
Flours	Barley flour, rye flour, buckwheat flour, potato flour, soya flour, cornflour, arrowroot flour, gluten-free flour, Terence Stamp's All Purpose Flour
Pasta	Rice noodles, corn pasta, buckwheat pasta, rice pasta shapes, barley pasta
Cereals	Porridge made from oats, barley, brown rice, millet, quinoa or buckwheat; cornflakes, puffed rice, wheat-free muesli, oat-based cereals, millet rice cereals
Breads	Rye bread (Village Bakery do some great ones – see Resources), German pumpernickel bread, sourdough bread, rice cakes and crackers, Ryvita, oatcakes, gluten-free breads available in healthfood shops

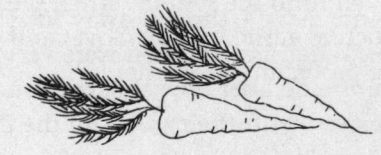

Dairy-free foods

Milk	Soya milk, oat milk, rice milk, coconut milk, almond milk
Butter	Dairy-free spreads such as Granose, Vitaquell and Vitaseig. For cooking, use extra-virgin olive oil. For baking, use unhydrogenated cooking margarine such as Vitaquell cuisine or unrefined sunflower oil
Yoghurt	Soya yoghurt (natural and fruit varieties are available), goat's and sheep's yoghurt (if tolerated)
Cheese	Soya cheese, goat's and sheep's cheeses (if tolerated)
Cream	Soya cream, cashew cream

For a healthy immune system – let them eat dirt

One in seven children in the UK now suffers from asthma, and the numbers are still rising. The latest and most probable theory is that we have become a hygiene-obsessed culture. We are now living in smaller family units, in highly insulated, cleaner homes, and children today are less exposed than previous generations to germs in the environment. There is unlikely to be a house in the country with young children which lacks a spray bottle of Dettox, wielded to clean tables, babies' high chairs, toys and so on.

But children need a healthy exposure to germs in order to build up their immune systems. I have never bathed my children every day, nor have I thrown away food the moment it falls on the floor. When my children were very young, and we lived in London, I remember how shocked some of my friends were that they played with their trucks in the flowerbeds. As it happens, there were very few flowers and so it made a perfect temporary alternative to a sandpit! A bit of dirt never hurt anybody, and in terms of your children's health it may be just what they need.

The ingredients of a healthy immune system

- Exercise
- Clean air
- Clean water
- Happiness
- Immune-boosting diet

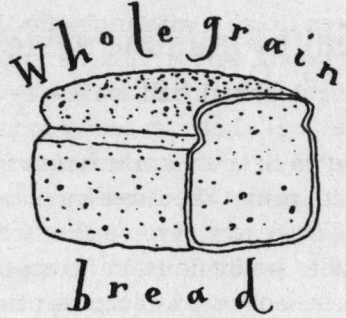

Chapter 3

•

ANTIBIOTICS–FRIEND OR FOE?

'FROM 2002, YOU COULD get a sore throat on a Tuesday, and be dead by Friday.' Since the 1950s the answer to any type of bacterial infection has been to zap it with antibiotics. In 1998 in the UK, 47 million prescriptions were written for antibiotics alone. But now the bugs are fighting back, and as a result we are seeing antibiotic-resistant 'superbugs' that may soon conquer us all. Some of these bugs develop special pumps which squirt out the antibiotics faster than they can get in. Others develop chemicals that are able to chop up penicillin, or grow thick walls that make it impossible for the antibiotics to penetrate them. It appears that the more antibiotics we use, both on ourselves and on animals, the faster the bugs are developing resistance.

For example, a bacteria called *Staphylococcus aureus* (SA) – one of the most infectious – now poses a serious problem in the treatment of hospital patients. In the 1940s penicillin was hailed as the miracle drug in the battle against SA, but within eighteen months the bacterium had become resistant to it. In 1959 methicillin, a new antibiotic, was introduced to kill SA. Eighteen months later that too had been defeated and MRSA (methicillin-resistant SA) had emerged. Nowadays vancomycin, our most powerful antibiotic, is used. These drug-resistant microbes are causing such a problem, especially in hospitals, that, according to the World Health Organization, 60 per cent of hospital infections are now caused by them. In the United States, 14,000 patients die every year from drug-resistant bacteria picked up in hospital.

It is not only the antibiotics that we take as medicines that are causing the problem. Farmed animals and fish are routinely given antibiotics to prevent disease and as growth promoters. The residues from these antibiotics are turning up in the meat and fish we eat and the milk we drink, and there is now evidence that cross-resistance from animal to human drugs may be occurring. For example, resistance to avoparcin, widely used in pig and poultry farming, may be transferring to vancomycin. In 1995, one particular strain of salmonella picked up on a farm was found to be resistant to five antibiotics.

If we continue to prescribe and use antibiotics at the current rate, more drug-resistant bacteria will emerge. Diseases once thought to be retreating are making a comeback. During the last ten years outbreaks of plague, diphtheria, yellow fever, meningitis, influenza and cholera have claimed many lives worldwide. According to the World Health Organization, over thirty new ones have emerged since the early 1980s. In terms of our long-term health we need to be more discriminating in the way we use antibiotics. They should never be given for a viral infection – such as a cold or flu – and should be used only to treat the specific bacterium in question. As far as children's health is concerned we need to find ways to bypass antibiotics unless absolutely necessary, and to use more natural ways of helping children fight off infections. If we do this, their immune systems will become stronger and more able to deal with whatever pathogenic (disease-causing) bacteria they do encounter.

Why antibiotics are bad for your child's immune system

Antibiotics work by killing bacteria. However, they are not discriminating about which bacteria they destroy and in the process many of those which we actually need in order to be healthy are killed off too. An amazing 30 per cent of faecal matter is made up of bacteria, some good and some bad. We live with just over a kilo (3 lb) of bacteria occupying our gut. The ratio between the bacteria that are health-promoting and those that are disease-provoking is determined by our lifestyles, stress levels, diet and any antibiotic therapy we are undergoing.

Let us look for a second at where these bacteria come from in terms of your child's development. Before birth, your baby has a sterile gut. During birth she will pick up bacteria from the birth canal and the environment. The development of her intestinal flora (bacteria) is then largely dependent on whether she is breast-fed or bottle-fed.

In breast-fed babies, Bifidobacteria quickly come to dominate their gastrointestinal tract. They produce acid faeces in a newborn baby and therefore inhibit the growth of harmful bacteria. The other bacteria in the gut of a newborn consist of lactobacilli (beneficial), enterococci and coliforms. If undisturbed, this community of bacteria will remain the same until the introduction of solid food, when the gut will start to develop a typical adult flora.

Bottle-fed babies develop a different gut flora. They contain mostly lactobacilli, but have far fewer Bifidobacteria and more significant levels of enterococci and coliforms. This imbalance is cited as one reason that bottle-fed babies are more susceptible to gastro-intestinal infection resulting in mild to severe diarrhoea. The good news is that bottle-fed babies can now be given Bifidobacteria supplements, which will help to restore the balance.

If your child takes in antibiotics, the balance of the gut

Why don't antibiotics work against viruses?

Very simply, bacteria are single-cell organisms. They contain a cell wall, a plasma membrane and a nucleus containing genetic material. Antibiotics work by damaging different parts of the cell and hence killing the bacteria (see page 21 on resistant bacteria).

Viruses, like the ones that cause colds, flu, measles and chicken pox, are not living cells. The do not have a cell wall or membrane. Therefore, since antibiotics cannot attack the structure of a virus, they are rendered useless against them.

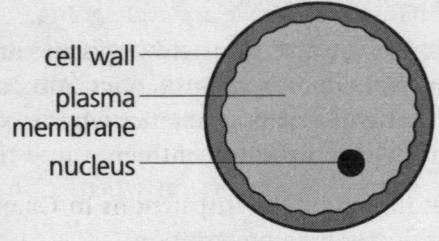

cell wall
plasma membrane
nucleus

**A bacteria
(highly simplified)**

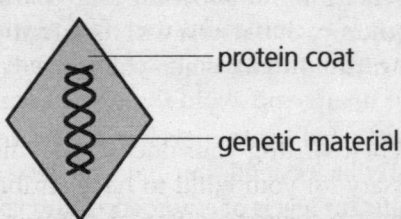

protein coat

genetic material

**A virus
(highly simplified)**

bacteria is disrupted – a large percentage of the good as well as the bad bacteria are wiped out. One course of antibiotics can wipe out beneficial strains of bacteria such as lactobacillus and Bifidobacteria for six months or more. These beneficial bacteria are called probiotics. They are part of your children's first line of defence against harmful bacteria, viruses and fungi, as well as other disease-producing microbes. They also produce important B vitamins, improve digestion, increase resistance to infection, and produce substances called bacteriocins which act as natural antibiotics to kill undesirable micro-organisms.

Six-step plan to avoid antibiotics

1. Put your family on an organic diet. Meat, fish, eggs and dairy products can all contain residues from antibiotics. Although organic animals can be treated with antibiotics when necessary, they are not routinely pumped full of them.

2. If your child does get ill, follow the instructions in Chapter 13 before asking your doctor for a prescription.

3. Make sure children rest when they are ill. Filling them with paracetamol and sending them off to school may be an easier option, but they are likely to come back feeling worse. Colds and flus are viral; it is normally a secondary infection that is bacterial and therefore treated with antibiotics. Treating the virus will help to prevent any bacterial infection occurring and avoid the need for antibiotics.

4. When visiting your doctor, ask whether it is absolutely necessary for your child to have antibiotics. You may find he or she can suggest a different solution.

5. Avoid all mucous-forming foods (mainly dairy products), since mucus is a breeding-ground for bacteria.

6. Give your child plenty of fluids in the form of diluted juices, water and juice boosts (see page 244).

Chapter 4

•

SUPER-IMMUNITY – ARE VACCINATIONS THE ANSWER?

ACCORDING TO THE World Health Organization, 'we are standing on the brink of a global crisis in infectious diseases. No country is safe from them. No country can any longer afford to ignore their threat. Of the 52 million deaths from all causes in 1995, more than 17 million were due to infectious diseases, including 9 million deaths in young children.'

Vaccinations have long been hailed as one of the miracles of modern science, and as we enter the third millennium ever-increasing numbers of vaccines are being formulated to protect our children from infectious diseases. These are basically diseases you can catch. They can either be transmitted from person to person, as in chicken pox, or from animal to person, as in rabies. Most infectious diseases are contracted through the intestinal tract or the respiratory system; rabies and tetanus, however, enter the body through a wound in the skin. The infectious diseases we hear most about today in relation to children are measles, mumps, meningitis, whooping cough, chicken pox and tuberculosis.

How do vaccinations work?

Immunity from a disease occurs naturally when, for example, a child catches an infectious disease such as measles. The child's immune system launches an assault on the virus, antibodies are formed and battle is joined. Once the infection is destroyed the child's symptoms disappear, leaving the antibodies to man the fortress to prevent any further invasion by the same enemy.

Vaccination is based on the belief that you can create the same immunity by inoculating either with ready-made antibodies or with live, killed or so-called harmless versions of the micro-organism, which will stimulate the immune system to launch a mini-assault and create antibodies. This is called artificial immunity. At present in the UK, children receive a massive twenty-four doses of vaccine by the time they go to school. Meningitis C is currently being added to the programme and will be fully incorporated by 2001.

To vaccinate or not to vaccinate – that is the question

Whether or not to vaccinate your child is one of the most emotive decisions that a parent has to make at the start of their baby's life. It is made no easier by the fact that the two sides are so fiercely in opposition. Enormous pressure is put on parents to vaccinate their children. Deciding not to is a huge responsibility. However, as vaccination is not compulsory in the UK, as it is in the United States, we do still have freedom of choice. To discuss this issue in depth would require a book in itself, but here is a quick overview of the controversy which will enable you to do some research before making that all-important 'informed decision'.

The current vaccination programme for UK children

Age	Vaccination	Method
2 months	Haemophilus influenza Type b (Hib), diptheria, tetanus, whooping cough (DPT) Polio	One injection By mouth
3 months	Haemophilus influenza Type b (Hib), diptheria, tetanus, whooping cough (DPT) Polio	One injection By mouth
4 months	Haemophilus influenza Type b (Hib), diptheria, tetanus, whooping cough (DPT) Polio	One injection By mouth
12–15 months	Measles, mumps and rubella (MMR)	Injection
3–5 years	Diptheria, tetanus Polio Measles, mumps and rubella (MMR)	Booster injection By mouth Booster injection
10–14 years	Tuberculosis (BCG)	Injection
13–18 years	Diptheria, tetanus Polio	Booster injection By mouth

The vaccine debate at a glance

For	Against
Vaccination is responsible for the decline in infectious diseases	Statistical evidence shows that diseases were well in decline before immunisation programmes were ever brought in. Better sanitation and improved diets were responsible
The benefits of vaccination far outweigh the risks	According to the Health Education Authority, 1 in 1,000 children will have a bad reaction to the MMR resulting in a fit (HEA, *From Birth to Five*). A study published in the *Lancet* in 1989 stated that the figure is more likely to be 1 in 400. The UK Vaccine Damage Payment Act was passed in 1979 to compensate those severely damaged by vaccinations. To date around £10 million has been paid out

For	Against
The vaccination will protect you against the disease	'The United States Center for Disease Control and Prevention has issued new guidelines for administering the polio vaccine after determining that nearly all the cases of paralytic polio contracted recently in the country were caused by the oral polio vaccine' (*British Medical Journal*, vol. 314, 15 February 1997)
The diseases you are vaccinated against are life-threatening	The diseases are only life-threatening in poorly nourished or chronically ill children. According to the UK Department of Health, out of eleven deaths in the UK due to measles in the previous nine years only four were due to acute measles illness itself and the others were due to neurological conditions (*Immunisation against Infectious Disease*, HMSO, 1996)
If the majority of a population are vaccinated, then everyone will be protected	In a 1986 outbreak of measles in Corpus Christi, Texas, 99 per cent of the children had been vaccinated (Walene James, *Immunization*, p.46)

Finding out more

One of the difficulties in making this decision is that no one knows the cocktail effect of our current immunisation programme. However, it is more likely that adverse reactions are going to occur in children whose immune systems are compromised. You are unlikely to know if there are any subtle immunodisorders that could be triggered in your child when she is only two months old. What is more, some of the diseases that our children our immunised against are not life-threatening in developed countries with well-nourished populations. Measles, mumps and whooping cough are common childhood diseases, which serve a purpose in immune development. As a group of Swedish doctors remarked in 1990, 'We have lost the common sense and the wisdom that used to prevail in the approach to childhood diseases. Too often, instead of reinforcing the organism's defences, fever and symptoms are relentlessly suppressed. This is not always without consequences . . . .'

To make your decision easier, spend some time reading about the pros and cons. Your health visitor will provide you with leaflets outlining the benefits of vaccination. The Department of Health produces a book called *Immunisation against Infectious Disease,* which is updated every four years (at the time of writing, the latest was 2000). It is obviously promotional but does contain a lot of information about consent, the diseases, side-effects and contra-indications. Your doctor's surgery should have a copy, as will most public libraries. What Doctors Don't Tell You produce *The WDDTY Vaccination Bible,* which is an easy-to-read, fully referenced guide to why you should consider not immunising your child. (For details of availability of these books see Resources.)

If you have access to the Internet there are endless websites regarding vaccination. The World Health Organization has an extensive site (www.who.ch) covering everything from present predictions on infectious diseases to an in-depth report and details of vaccines in development, as well as the most commonly asked questions and answers to them.

An organisation called The Informed Parent was set up in the UK in 1992. Membership is on an annual basis with a quarterly newsletter, a comprehensive reading list containing videos and audio tapes, and details of talks and meetings on vaccination. See Resources for a more extensive reading list.

The four options

In my practice I am frequently asked my opinion on vaccinations, and my answer is that you can only decide when you have looked at both sides of the argument. No one else can decide for you. However, the decision has to be made at a time when you are feeling emotionally vulnerable, and some mothers really can't face thinking of anything other than the next feed.

In my opinion, there are four options to consider at this time:

1. Fully vaccinate your child and stick to the programme set out by the government

2. Partially vaccinate your child, avoiding the most controversial ones such as whooping cough (pertussis) and MMR (that decision can wait until your child is a year old)

3. Postpone the programme for a few months until you feel strong enough to consider it

4. Don't vaccinate your child at all

What's the alternative to vaccination?

Deciding not to vaccinate your child is a huge responsibility. If it is the choice you propose to make then you must be prepared to take full responsibility for your child's health, putting into practice all the measures outlined in the following chart in order to keep her immune system fighting fit

---

Super-immunity without vaccination

- Breast-feed your baby for as long as possible. If you can, do so exclusively for the first six months while your baby's immune system is finding its own feet. While you are breast-feeding eat a nutrient-rich organic diet and take a multi-vitamin and mineral designed for breast-feeding mothers.

- When you are weaning your baby on to solids, make sure her diet is rich in immune-boosting nutrients (vitamins A, C and E,

continues ▶

selenium, zinc, iron, calcium, magnesium and potassium). The 1999 WHO report on infectious diseases claimed that in developing countries, 'As many as one in four child deaths from infectious diseases – mainly from measles and diarrhoea – could be prevented by giving children vitamin A supplements.' This shows just how important nutrients are. In the developed world, however, a diet rich in beta-carotene, a precursor of vitamin A (which means the body can convert beta-carotene into vitamin A) is the best defence.

- Avoid giving your child processed and refined foods or those containing preservatives, flavours and artificial colourings, which are all immune-suppressive. Wherever possible use wholegrains, which have a higher nutrient content. Look in your larder, and if it's white throw it out!

- Use herbal remedies such as echinacea, garlic, tea tree and elderberry, and nutritional supplements such as vitamin C and zinc, to help combat infections.

- Only allow antibiotics to be prescribed when there is no other option, and never for viral infections (against which they will not work).

- Take your baby to a homeopath at two months for constitutional treatment and homeopathic nosodes (tablets or drops) against the diseases (see Resources for a local homeopath).

- Make sure your child drinks pure, clean water and gets lots of fresh air and exercise, all of which will help to boost the immune system.

- Don't be obsessed with cleanliness: exposure to a little dirt helps to prime a child's immune system.

continues ►

- Keep your children at home as babies and avoid day care, which is a breeding ground for infections.

- Be aware of the symptoms of meningitis – pinprick rash, stiff neck, fever, vomiting, severe headache and difficulty with bright lights – and if you suspect it rush your child to hospital immediately. If it is caught in time, doctors could save her life.

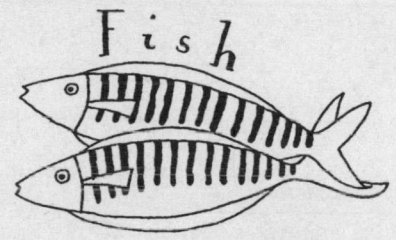

PART TWO

·

The Immune Boosting Diet

The following chapters explain how to
prepare the best foods for your child and
give her the right nutrients. From baby's first
purées to healthy teenage snacks, there are
plenty of tasty immune-boosting recipes
for all the family.

Chapter 5

•

THE ESSENTIAL HEALTHY DIET

Even before your baby is born, you are able to enhance the development of her immune system. While you are pregnant, the nutrients in the foods you are eating nourish your baby. The strength of your baby's immune system depends a great deal on the supply and quality of these nutrients. Your baby also gains immune protection through your own antibodies, which are transferred across the placenta during pregnancy.

Once born, your baby will continue to be protected by your antibodies for the first few months of her life; after that her immune system will be sufficiently mature to start manufacturing its own. Breast-feeding your baby is another important immune-enhancer. Breast milk contains nutrients and special substances that can directly protect your baby against infection and allergies (see page 79).

Delaying weaning until six months is yet another wonderful way of helping to build a strong immune system for your baby. At this age, your baby's intestines will be sufficiently mature to cope with the introduction of foods and will have received a good protective layer of beneficial bacteria through your breast milk.

Once your baby is weaned, there is a powerful immune-boosting diet that you can introduce her to. In the age of the 'superbug', increasing numbers of new diseases and escalating allergies, we need to look to nature for the nutrients required to build healthy, strong children, and to use natural anti-microbial agents which can assist the immune system and kill bugs and viruses that threaten our children's health.

Whatever age your children are, the food that they eat will directly affect their health. In past centuries sailors who undertook long voyages without supplies of fresh fruit and vegetables developed scurvy, the vitamin C deficiency disease. In the same way undernourished children, too, will develop deficiency symptoms. Feeding them on an immune-boosting diet will supply them with all the nutrients they need to keep them healthy all year round.

The top ten immune-boosting nutrients

To build children with super-resistance, we need to feed them food packed with immune-boosting nutrients. Here are the top ten vitamins and minerals which help to build immunity and protect your children against disease and allergies. Foods in which these nutrients are found are listed in the table on page 45. The body parts and functions mentioned below were described in Chapter 1.

Vitamin A

This fat-soluble vitamin acts as a powerful antioxidant (see page 46) as well as helping to metabolise essential fatty acids (see page 47). It is required for maintaining an active thymus gland, and therefore for B- and T-cell maturation. It is also involved in maintaining the mucous membranes of the respiratory, urinary and digestive systems. Liver is an excellent source but, since this vitamin is fat-soluble, too much can be toxic. So only give liver to a child once a week, maximum.

Beta-carotene

The body converts beta-carotene into retinol, the active form of vitamin A. As the body can regulate this conversion rate, your child will not make more than she needs and beta-carotene can therefore not become toxic.

B-complex

The B vitamins B1, B2, B3, B5, B6, B12 and folic acid work together and are important for immune health. B6 and B3 help EFAs convert into anti-inflammatory prostaglandins. B6 is also needed for the function of the phagocytic cells. B5 is required for antibody production as well as making sure the immune army of white cells can do their job effectively.

Vitamin C

This, the king of immune-boosting nutrients, is antibacterial and antiviral as well as being a powerful antioxidant. It is a natural antihistamine, which helps with the body's response to allergens, and the body also requires it for EFA metabolism. As it is water-soluble, vitamin C is safe to use in supplemental form for babies and toddlers in response to infection. For information on dosage see Chapter 13.

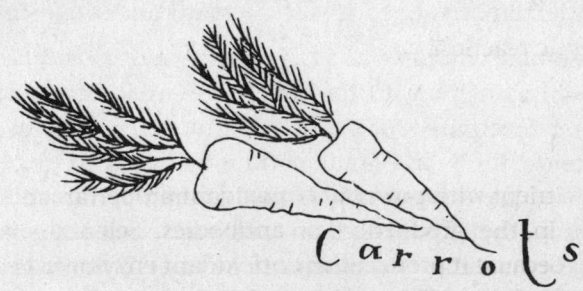

Carrots

Vitamin E

Another fat-soluble vitamin which the body can store, vitamin E is an antioxidant which helps to protect tissues from damage caused by pollution. It is also needed for an efficient antibody response to infection.

Iron

This mineral is vital for your child's immune system. It is also the nutrient that is frequently low in toddlers and teenagers, causing anaemia. Iron is needed for the production of white blood cells and antibodies, and without sufficient iron your child is more likely to suffer from frequent colds and infections. Eating vitamin C-rich foods at the same meal as iron-rich foods will enhance the absorption of the iron.

Zinc

This mineral promotes the growth and development of your child's white blood cells, especially the lymphocytes. It also helps to keep the thymus healthy and active. It is a powerful antioxidant and is also involved in EFA metabolism. Unfortunately, zinc is commonly deficient in children. Although one of the best sources is shellfish, as these are shoreline creatures they are at high risk of pollution. Check your source of supply carefully, and remember not to give shellfish to under-twos in case of an allergic reaction.

Selenium

Another nutrient with powerful antioxidant properties, this mineral helps in the production of antibodies. Selenium is also important because it produces an antioxidant enzyme called glutathione peroxidase. The soil in the UK contains low selenium levels, so it is important to include good sources of natural selenium in our daily diet. Seafood is a good source but see the note under Zinc, above.

Calcium

Although best known for its effect on bones and teeth, calcium is also important for efficient functioning of the immune system. It is also required to operate the complement system (see page 7), and by all phagocytic cells if they are to function correctly. EFA metabolism is also dependent on calcium, among other nutrients.

Magnesium

Yet another very important mineral for immune health, magnesium is also frequently deficient in people who live in the UK. It is needed for the metabolism of EFAs. It is also required for antibody production. Low levels of magnesium can increase allergic reactions. This is because a deficiency of magnesium can cause histamine levels to rise.

Antioxidant protection – the vital nutrients

An antioxidant is a nutrient that protects the cells in the body from oxidative damage. Oxidation occurs when a substance reacts with oxygen, for example when an apple, a banana or an avocado are cut and exposed to the air and turns brown. An antioxidant can prevent or at least diminish this process which is why we squeeze lemon or lime juice (which contain the antioxidant vitamin C) on these fruit. Your child's cells use oxygen all the time for the process of combustion: to burn food for energy production, and to get rid of germs and foreign chemicals such as pesticides. During this process, substances called

Immune-boosting vitamins and minerals – which foods contain what?

Vitamins and minerals	Best sources (organic where possible)
Vitamin A	Liver, eggs, full-fat dairy products, cod liver oil, oily fish like herring and mackerel
Beta-carotene water	Butternut squash, pumpkin, cantaloupe melon, melon, carrots, sweet potatoes, apricots, mangoes, green leafy vegetables
B-complex vitamins	Wholegrains, liver, poultry, game, wheatgerm
Vitamin C	Broccoli, parsley, kiwi fruit, citrus fruit, berries, peppers (capsicums), blackcurrants, Brussels sprouts, papaya, mangoes
Vitamin E	Avocados, nuts, seeds, unrefined oils, wheatgerm, oatmeal
Iron	Liver, red meat, eggs, wholegrains, green leafy vegetables beans, lentils, nuts, seeds, blackstrap molasses
Zinc	Shellfish, poultry (especially dark meat), game, lean red meat, pulses, seeds (especially pumpkin), nuts, wholegrains
Selenium	Nuts (especially brazil), seeds (especially sesame), wholegrains, seafood
Calcium	Dairy products, fortified soya products, nuts (especially almonds) seeds, tinned fish with bones e.g. salmon and sardines, dark green vegetables like broccoli and kale
Magnesium	Nuts, seeds, green leafy vegetables, root vegetables, egg yolks, wholegrains, dried fruit

free radicals are formed which can cause cellular damage and can trigger disease.

Free radicals are produced by all forms of combustion. Environmental pollution is another major source, as well as smoking, radiation and browned and burnt foods such as barbecued foods. Fried foods contain plenty of free radicals as the high heat damages the oil. Fast food restaurants are a disaster area for young immune systems, as children consume copious amounts of heat-damaged oils washed down with a fat-laden milkshake or sugar-filled fizzy drink. Luckily nature is armed with rich sources of antioxidant nutrients that are capable of disarming free radicals. Your child will need a diet rich in antioxidants all her life, so here is where to find them.

Antioxidants – which foods contain what?

Antioxidant	Best sources (organic where possible)
Vitamin A	Liver, eggs, cod liver oil, full-fat dairy products
Beta-carotene	Butternut squash, pumpkin, cantaloupe melon, water melon, carrot, sweet potatoes, apricots, green leafy vegetables
Vitamin C	Broccoli, parsley, kiwi fruit, citrus fruit, berries, peppers (capsicums), blackcurrants, Brussels sprouts, papaya, mangoes
Vitamin E	Avocados, nuts, seeds, unrefined oils, wheatgerm, oatmeal
Zinc	Shellfish, poultry (especially dark meat), game, lean red meat, pulses, seeds (especially pumpkin), nuts, wholegrains
Selenium	Nuts (especially brazil), seeds (especially sesame), wholegrains, seafood

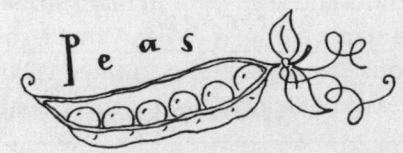

Phytonutrients

As more research into health is conducted, an ever-increasing number of compounds found in food are discovered to have powerful health-promoting properties. These components are not classed as essential to life like vitamins and minerals, but they do appear to be hugely beneficial to our health. For example, it is common knowledge that oranges are rich in vitamin C, but they are also a rich source of hesperidin, a bioflavonoid with antioxidant properties which works synergistically with vitamin C and increases the potential of the vitamin. Over a hundred phytonutrients have so far been identified, many of them possessing powerful immune-boosting properties. Preparing foods that are rich in the natural colours red, orange, green, yellow, purple and blue will ensure that you and your child receive plenty of these beneficial nutrients. See the table on page 48.

Essential fatty acids (EFAs) and your child's immune system

Conclusive research has shown that the amount and type of fat consumed during foetal development, infancy, childhood, adolescence and even adulthood have a profound effect on our health. British children eat far too much saturated fat and not nearly enough of the right type of polyunsaturated fats which contain health-promoting substances and essential fatty acids (EFAs). As the body is unable to convert other fats into essential fatty acids, these fats have to come directly from the food we eat. EFAs are found in many foods, but are most abundant in the oils of certain nuts and seeds and in oily fish. Sadly, these foods are no longer a staple part of our diet. What is more, if your children have a poor diet filled with saturated fat they are unlikely to be able to assimilate whatever little essential fat they do consume.

There are two main families of essential fatty acids, omega-3 and omega-6. In the presence of certain vitamins and minerals they are converted into prostaglandins, hormone-like sub- stances which, amongst other things, regulate the activity of white blood cells. They are therefore vital to the functioning of your child's immune system. Without adequate essential fatty acids your child will be more prone to colds, infections and allergies.

One extremely efficient way of making sure your child has plenty of essential fatty acids is to supplement her diet with oils rich in these nutrients. Whilst you are breast-feeding your baby

Natural colour – which foods contain what?

Colour	Phytonutrient	Properties	Good food source
Red	Lycopene	Antioxidant	Tomatoes
Yellow	Curcumin	Antioxidant	English mustard, corn, yellow peppers
	Anthoxanthins	Antioxidants	Yellow-skinned onions, potatoes
Orange	Carotenoids	Antioxidants essential in maintaining an active immune system	Carrots, squashes, mangoes, sweet papaya, apricots, cantaloupe melon
Blue/ purple/red	Anthocyanidins and proanthocyanidins Quercetin	Antioxidants Antioxidant which is involved in the body's regulation, synthesis and release of certain cells called leukotrienes	Blueberries, purple grapes, blackberries, black cherries, blackcurrants, beetroot, cranberries, onions, apples immune
Green	Chlorophyll	Protects against cancer, good wound healer	Wheat grass, algae, seaweed, green vegetables such as broccoli, kale and cabbage, salad leaves

The lowdown on fats

Fat is a necessary component of our bodies:

- It keeps us warm
- It keeps our skin and arteries supple
- It is essential for proper brain function
- It is a source of energy
- It cushions our internal organs

But there are different kinds of fat and some are much better for us than others.

Type	Where found	For	Against
Saturated	Butter, hard cheeses, palm and coconut oil, fatty meats	Eat in moderation	Too much increases risk of heart disease and encourages inflammatory conditions e.g. asthma, eczema, arthritis
Trans fats	Hydrogenated margarines (formed by converting vegetable oil into fat at very high temperatures). Used in commercially produced cakes, pies, biscuits and crisps	Not beneficial to your child's health	Contributes to heart disease and cancer
Unsaturated (two types with slightly different chemical compositions)			
(1) Monounsaturated	Olive oil, rapeseed oil, avocados, nuts, seeds	Olive is the best oil for cooking because heating does not cause it to produce dangerous free radicals (see page 46)	
(2) Polyunsaturated	Seeds, nuts (and their oils, e.g. sunflower, safflower), oily fish (e.g. salmon, mackerel)	This group includes EFAs omega-3 and omega-6, vital for immune function and brain development	When heated they form free radicals, believed to contribute to heart disease and cancer

will be receiving plenty of EFAs, as breast milk is a marvellous source. Once she is off the breast and on to solids, add one teaspoon of flaxseed oil a day to her food or bottle. Flaxseed (linseed) oil is a great source of omega-3. To ensure she gets enough omega-6 pierce an evening primrose oil capsule and rub it into her tummy once a day. This is especially beneficial if there are allergies in the family. Babies over one year old can be given a specially formulated blend of oils which has the ideal ratio of omega-3 and omega-6 (see Resources).

Good and bad fat sources at a glance

Good	Bad
Flaxseeds (linseeds) and flaxseed oil	Eggs
	Butter
Walnuts and walnut oil	Cream
Hemp and hemp oil	Cheese
Soya beans and soya bean oil	Beef, lamb, pork
Sunflower seeds	Roasted nuts and seeds
Pumpkin seeds	Refined oils
Sesame seeds	Hydrogenated margarines
Fresh oily fish from unpolluted waters	Lard and shortenings
Evening primrose oil	Heat-damaged oils found in chips, crisps and other fried and deep-fried foods

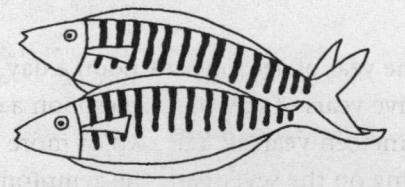

Does your child have an EFA deficiency?

If your child has three or more of the symptoms below, she may be lacking in EFAs. Supplement her diet with an oil blend for a month and see if her symptoms improve (see recipe for Essential Fatty Acid Tonic on page 247).

Here are the symptoms to look out for:

- Dry skin
- Red pimples on back of arms
- Alligator (scaly) skin
- Cracked skin
- Eczema
- Poor wound healing
- Dry hair
- Dandruff
- Brittle nails
- Excessive thirst
- Irritability
- Frequent urination
- Hyperactivity
- Attention deficit disorder
- Learning problems
- Frequent colds and infections
- Allergies
- Lowered immunity
- Tiredness and weakness

Dosage
- up to one year of age: one teaspoon a day
- one to five years of age: one tablespoon a day
- six to nineteen years of age: two or more tablespoons a day, depending on the severity of the symptoms

Water – is your child drinking enough?

Some 70 per cent of your child's body consists of water, and she cannot live more than a few days without it. Water has enormous health-promoting qualities: it stops the lymphatic system getting sluggish, improves circulation and boosts concentration.

Yet research in 1995 from Southampton University has shown that most children do not drink enough water. One of our most important nutrients has become totally overlooked. Tea, coffee, fizzy drinks, squashes and fruit drinks are no substitute because they contain undesirable substances such as sugar and caffeine, and some of them actually dehydrate the body. To function efficiently, your child's body needs water. So how do you know that she is drinking enough of it?

One of the best lessons that you can teach your child is to notice the colour of her urine. Before you shriek with laughter, this was not a lesson that I can take credit for instigating in my family. It was my eldest son's first school teacher, Caroline Tuffnell, who taught him that if his 'wee' was dark yellow he was not drinking enough. It needed to be a very pale yellow. Clever her – she is one of the first teachers I have met who has made the connection between brain output and dietary input. What is more, my son now has a useful reminder to drink more!

Why do children appear to dislike water so much? If you live in London (and many other places too) I'm sure you know the answer already. What comes out of our taps tastes disgusting. Therefore we add things to disguise it and make it more palatable.

But it is possible to make water taste better without adding flavourings. A jug filter is cheap and removes most of the nasty-tasting components, such as chlorine, as well as some other undesirables. If you want to take one step further, you can get a (rather more expensive) plumbed-in water filter (see Resources).

How to get your children to drink more water

- As soon as they get up offer them a drink of fresh juice, diluted 50/50 with water, warm or cold, whichever they prefer. This may seem a bore, but you are giving their bodies a wonderful start to the day. Once they are distracted with breakfast they will forget to drink.

- In the car, always have beakers of water or sports-type water bottles (available from supermarkets).

- Offer your children lots of raw fruit and vegetables as snacks. These contain lots of water and are therefore great substitutes.

- In hot weather, offer water more frequently.

- Drink water yourself!

- Offer water at one meal every day. My children always have water at teatime and drink it quite happily.

- Babies do not need baby juices. Give them water instead. Baby juices are mostly made up from water, colourings and sugar.

- Have water by your children's beds, in feeder cups or beakers. Children can get thirsty at night.

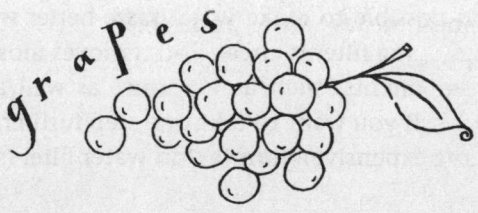

The immune-boosting diet – the complete jigsaw

So what should your child's diet look like overall to build a strong immune system? Balance is the key. The four basic building blocks of your child's diet are:

- water
- complex carbohydrates
- proteins
- fat

While you are breast-feeding, your baby is getting the perfect combination of all these elements in just one food. Once she is eating solid food, this slowly takes over as her main source of these building blocks. Here is a guide to the ideal immune-boosting diet for your child.

- **Your child's diet should be made up of:**
  - 50–65 per cent complex carbohydrates
  - 15–25 per cent proteins
  - 20–25 per cent fats

In real terms, let's look at how this converts into food intakes in a day.

- **Your child needs four to nine servings of complex carbohydrates a day. These include:**
  - wholemeal breads, pastas and cereals
  - brown rice
  - oats
  - barley
  - rye
  - corn

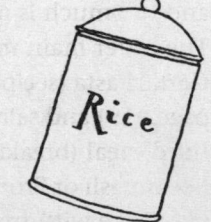

- millet
- buckwheat
- pulses
- potatoes

● **Your child needs five servings of fruit and vegetables a day.** These should include:
  - one leafy green vegetable such as broccoli, kale, spinach or dark green salad leaves (such as watercress, rocket, lollo and baby cos lettuces, herbs)
  - one orange fruit or vegetable such as carrot or orange
  - a purple, blue or red fruit or vegetable such as tomato, beetroot or some seasonal berries (even tomato ketchup will do as it contains plenty of lycopene. Choose a healthy brand (see Resources))
  - a root vegetable such as potato, parsnip, turnip, swede or beetroot
  - a watery vegetable or fruit such as lettuce, melon, berries, citrus fruit or kiwi fruit.

Shockingly, two-thirds of sixteen- to twenty-four-year-olds eat fruit less than once a week. Get good habits established when they are young.

● **Your child needs three to five servings of protein a day.** Every meal should contain some protein but only one meal a day should contain meat or fish – these are dense proteins, and too much is unnecessary and may overburden her body. The other main meal could be vegetarian like Courgette and Garlic Pasta (see page 169) or Baked Potato and Hummus (see page 119) and salad or Quick Nut Burgers (see page 206). The third meal (breakfast) could contain some nuts and/or seeds like muesli or Protein-packed Porridge (see page 137), or a liquid shake with fruit and yoghurt or tofu (see page 196).

- **Your child's liquid requirement is 1–3 pints (0.5–2.0 litres) a day** depending on her age and the weather. Starting the day off with diluted fresh juice (see page 53) is a marvellous way of rehydrating your child's body before breakfast.

- **Fats are essential to your child's diet**, but the trick is to ensure that you are providing enough of the good ones. Nuts, seeds and oily fish are packed full of essential fatty acids. To make doubly sure, supplement your child's diet daily with between one teaspoon and two tablespoons (depending on age) of a cold-pressed seed oil or oil blend (see EFAs on page 47). Cook with a little butter or extra-virgin olive oil. On bread and toast use an unhydrogenated spread such as Granose or Vitaquell. Salad dressings can be made with olive oil or cold-pressed safflower, sunflower or sesame oils.

For immune-boosting menu plans, look at the end of each age group section in Chapters 7–12.

The top five foods to avoid

As well as the food groups and individual foods that are good to include in your child's diet, there are also some which are better to do without wherever possible.

Sugar

Because sugar is a major immune suppressor it should not be part of an immune-boosting diet. As little as 100g (3½ oz) of sugar can suppress your child's immune system by up to 50 per cent. The American Journal of Clinical Nutrition published research as early as 1973 that showed that these effects start within half an hour of consuming sugar and can last up to five hours. Sucrose (white sugar) is devoid of nutrients. What is more, it actually requires nutrients for its metabolism and therefore will rob them from your child's body. Sugar in different guises is often hidden in foods specifically designed for young children. Most commercial baby food manufacturers use sugar in their ranges. The only one I have found that does not use sugar at all is Baby Organix. After the baby stage, foods specifically designed and marketed for children should be avoided wherever possible. In May 2000 a report by the Food Commission revealed that 57 per cent of the 358 children's foods they examined contained high levels of sugar. In one type of children's yoghurt there was five teaspoons of sugar in every pot. When looking at food labels in the supermarket, remember that a teaspoon of sugar is equivalent to 4g. Once you know this you can easily work out how many teaspoons of sugar are in any product. It will undoubtedly influence your food choices.

Hidden sugar

What's in a name? Look out for any of these on food labels: sucrose, glucose, glucose syrup, maltose, dextrose, inverted sugar syrup, lactose, golden syrup, honey, corn syrup, treacle, hydrolysed starch, fructose, concentrated fruit juice.

Salt

The Food Commission report also found raised salt levels in 46 per cent of the products tested. Salt is not allowed to be added to baby foods, but many children are given adult foods when they are very young. Babies and young children should not be eating crisps, savoury snacks, sausages, ham, bacon or smoked foods, which are too high in salt. Excess salt puts undue pressure on their kidneys, so that nutrients such as magnesium which are vital for a healthy immune system will be lost while their bodies deal with the salt. High salt intake also increases our risk of cardiovascular disease in later life. One breakfast cereal, Oat Krunchies, which claims to contain 100 per cent natural ingredients, has more salt in it than ready salted crisps – 1.1g per 100g. To protect your children's immune system and their overall health, you have to become an avid label watcher.

Hydrogenated fat

The process of hydrogenation involves turning a liquid oil into a solid or semi-solid margarine by affecting its chemical structure. This is done at extremely high temperatures and under pressure, which damages the oils and destroys their nutritional value. These types of fat also interfere with the metabolism of essential fatty acids. Hydrogenated fat is found not only in margarines but also in some biscuits, crisps, pastries and pies.

Caffeine

Many people think of caffeine as an undesirable substance found in coffee, but it is also present in tea, chocolate and chocolate drinks, as well as in fizzy drinks such as cola and Lucozade. Caffeine is a potent stimulant. It is also a powerful anti-nutrient that prevents your child's immune system getting the prostaglandins it needs. The 1995 Diet and Nutrition in Preschool Children survey reported that a staggering one-third of children under four and a half years of age were drinking tea.

If you have teenagers or even toddlers who are hooked on caffeine in one form or another, make some simple changes. Fizzy soft drinks can be swapped for similar but fruit-based ones such as Appletise and Aqua Libra, and tea and coffee can become decaffeinated until you decide you can get rid of them altogether. It is always easier and more proactive to add alternatives before taking the culprits away. For teenagers get a big selection of fruit teas, which tend to be the most popular of the herbal variety. Hot blackcurrant tea is delicious with a little raw honey drizzled into it. On a hot summer's day, soak three bags of blackcurrant fruit tea in a jug of boiling water for half an hour. Then remove the tea bags and allow the drink to cool. Add honey to taste and lots of crushed ice.

Additives

By avoiding most processed foods you will be saving your child from the chemical onslaught of additives in our food today. These additives come in the guises of:

- colourings
- flavourings
- emulsifiers
- stabilisers
- thickeners

- artificial sweeteners
- preservatives
- flavour enhancers
- glazing agents
- and many miscellanous additives

They are designed to make the food look good, taste good and last longer. There are now roughly 400 additives which can legally be included in our food, as well as over 3,500 substances used as flavours which do not even have to be listed on a label. These additives may put an unnecessary burden on your child's immune system, especially on the liver which is the primary site of detoxification. Foods and drinks specially prepared for babies and young children (essentially baby food, formula and baby drinks) are not allowed to contain certain additives. However, that does not include standard foods frequently eaten by small children such as savoury snacks, fizzy drinks, crisps, puddings, sausages, fish fingers, ice cream and sweets, which are packed full of these banned additives.

Avoiding additives – a quick guide

- Avoid processed meats such as sausages, bacon, ham and salami, or choose organic varieties.

- Avoid squashes and fruit drinks. Replace them with water or diluted fresh juice.

- Avoid packet and tinned foods, which are laced with additives.

- Avoid ready meals whenever you can, because they require many more additives to give them an extended shelf life.

- Eat foods in their most natural state. A roast chicken is a better choice than a processed chicken nugget, even if not quite as quick to prepare.

Preparing food safely for the family

In 1999 reported cases of food poisoning topped the 100,000 mark in the UK. But experts believe this is only the tip of the iceberg. It has been estimated that perhaps half a million people, many of them children, are affected by food poisoning every year.

The main culprits are:

- Campylobacter
- *E. coli*
- Listeria
- Salmonella
- *Bacillus cereus*
- Botulism
- *Staphylococcus aureus*

The bugs that cause food poisoning

Campylobacter

This is now the most commonly reported type of food poisoning, with the number of cases having doubled between the beginning and the end of the 1990s. The government believe that for every reported case of campylobacter poisoning, eight go unreported. The bacteria cause such severe stomach pains that they can be mistaken for appendicitis. Poultry, meat, shellfish and doorstep milk which has been pecked by birds can all carry the bacteria, which can also be caught from household pets.

Escherichia coli (E. coli)

E. coli can be found in the guts of both children and adults. Most types are harmless, but some can cause severe food poisoning and even death. Until the early 1990s food poisoning from *E. coli* was rare, but its incidence has since increased dramatically. It is commonly associated with undercooked meats, especially beef products such as burgers, and can also be found in unpasteurised milk and cheeses. Inadequate hygiene can contaminate meat in slaughterhouses and cause cross-contamination in butchers' shops.

Listeria

Listeria monocytogenes is found in soft ripened cheeses such as Brie and Camembert, pâtés, cold ready cooked meals and ice cream, especially the soft whip variety from machines. It is particularly dangerous to pregnant women as it can cause miscarriage, stillbirth or premature labour. The main problem with listeria is that it can still thrive at temperatures below 5°C (41°F).

Salmonella

Some years ago there was a dramatic increase in salmonella poisoning, which led to people being advised not to eat raw or undercooked eggs or foods containing them. Poultry and eggs are the main source of infection, but cooked foods or salads left unrefrigerated for several hours are also likely offenders. There is now evidence that some strains of salmonella have become antibiotic-resistant.

Bacillus cereus

This bacterium is found in cooked rice which has been kept warm or inadequately reheated. Cooked rice should be eaten straightaway or else cooled quickly and refrigerated. *Bacillus cereus* causes severe vomiting within one hour of eating, or diarrhoea later on, but recovery is rapid.

Clostridium botulinum (botulism)

This is a very rare form of food poisoning. The bacterium is found in poorly sterilised tinned or bottled fish, meat or vegetables.

Staphylococcus aureus

Most people carry this bacterium and it can easily be transferred to foods. Common culprits are ham, poultry and cream- or custard-filled baked goods.

Cooking equipment

For the recipes in this book, you will need very little high-tech gadgetry. In fact, you only need a few pieces of equipment (and if funds are limited you can improvise alternatives – see 'Cutting the cost . . .', page 64):

- **Food processor.** I use a Magimix, which has attachments for grating and slicing and a little bowl which fits in the middle and is perfect for blending instant meals for a baby.

● **Set of cups and spoons.** These days most supermarkets stock American cup sets and a spoon set ranging from teaspoon to tablespoon. These make cooking much easier and mean that many of my recipes do not require 'formal' measurements. I find that using a teacup, for example, does not work nearly as

---

Food preparation tips

When preparing food it is important to remember that babies and young children are more susceptible to food poisoning than adults, so proper hygiene in the kitchen is a must. Here are some healthy tips on food preparation to protect your whole family from infection.

● Wash your hands thoroughly before preparing food.

● Use a separate chopping board for meat, fish and poultry. Never cut bread, vegetables or fruit on this board.

● Always store cooked and raw food separately in the fridge. Cooked foods should be stored above raw meat so that meat juices cannot drip on to them and cause cross-contamination.

● Defrost meat and fish thoroughly before cooking.

● Make sure all foods are cooked thoroughly.

● Wash fruit and vegetables thoroughly, especially if they are going to be eaten raw. Peel fruit if it is not organic, as this will protect your children from pesticide residues.

● Eat leftovers within two days, and don't reheat food more than once.

● Keep your fridge at the correct temperature, which is 5°C (41°F). The freezer should be set at minus 18°C (0°F). Frozen foods should be thoroughly defrosted before use and not refrozen.

well as having the real things – and they are cheap, which is a bonus.

- **Steamer.** This is marvellous for cooking all vegetables and for cooking purées for a baby, especially when you want them to be a bit thicker than normal.

- **Ice cube trays and freezer bags.** These are invaluable for making and freezing baby purées.

- **Juicer.** The king of juicers is the Champion Juicer. It fulfils many functions, prepares unbeatable juices, and I am a complete convert. It is, unfortunately, incredibly expensive and you may prefer to start with one of the many smaller juicers that are widely available in department stores.

Cutting the cost of an immune-boosting diet for your family

If you want to feed your family an immune-boosting diet on a tight budget, here are some useful tips:

- Use an organic fruit and vegetable box scheme (see Resources) but get the delivery every other week instead of every week. Some are very reasonable

- Make leftover vegetables into soup which can feed the whole family for another meal

- Reduce the amount of meat you feed your family and increase vegetable protein (like pulses, grains and vegetables), which is much cheaper

- Instead of buying a steamer, use a colander over a pan and put a lid on top

- Use a hand blender instead of a food processor

- Buy organic meat and fish in bulk and freeze

- Menu plan at the beginning of the week, before you do the shopping, to avoid unnecessary food wastage

- Never buy speculatively, only what you know you need

- Use seasonal fruit and vegetables

- If you have a local market, visit it at the end of market day and you will be surprised at the bargains you can strike, even with organic market sellers!

- Visit the Internet for the best deals around

- Try not to buy commercialised products, such as Star Wars yoghurts! They cost more than ordinary ones.

Freezing safely

Making, freezing and serving baby foods

Peel and chop your fruit or vegetables and place them in the steamer or steamer substitute. Cook until soft, then purée until smooth. Sterilise ice cube trays by pouring boiling water over them (the type called Twist and Out are the easiest from which to extract frozen baby food cubes). Scoop the purées into the ice cube trays, smooth the surface with a knife, cover and allow to cool. Once cooled, place in the freezer until frozen hard. Then twist the cubes out of the trays and place them in freezer bags labelled with the date on which they were made, so that you do not give your baby out-of-date frozen food.

To serve a meal from the freezer for your baby, remove the relevant number of food cubes from the freezer and allow them to defrost at room temperature, covered with a tea towel. A fruit or vegetable purée may only take an hour or two to defrost, whereas a mixed meal of fish or meat and vegetables may take several hours. Make sure all food is completely thawed before heating. Once defrosted, heat the food gently in a pan, and cool before offering it to your baby. Do not reheat foods more than once and never refreeze uneaten food.

Freezing times

Your freezer should be set at minus 18°C (0°F)

- Fruit purées   3 months
- Vegetable purées   3 months
- Meat, cooked   3 months
- Fish, cooked   2 months
- Pulses and grains 2 months

Cooking methods for strong immune systems

Any form of cooking inevitably results in the loss of some nutrients, which is why a high percentage of raw food in your child's diet is the best way of ensuring a correspondingly high intake of antioxidant nutrients. The best cooking methods are as follows:

Grilling or griddling

This is very useful for cooking fish and lean meat as it uses so much less fat than frying.

Steaming

This is an excellent way of protecting vegetables and other foods from nutrient loss. Broccoli, for example, can lose over 60 per cent of its vitamin C when boiled but only 20 per cent when steamed. Vegetables cooked 'al dente' rather than until soft taste much nicer and will retain even more nutrients. The only time it is necessary to cook vegetables until really soft is when you are preparing baby purées.

Baking

Another good cooking method, baking uses less fat than roasting or frying. But don't wrap food in foil to cook it. Aluminium, now known to be a potentially toxic metal, can leach out of the foil into the food. It is much better to place the food in an oven-ware dish and then cover it with the foil, so that they are not actually touching.

Stir-frying

This is another way of retaining vital nutrients as only a very little oil is used and the vegetables are very lightly cooked. If you have children who loathe vegetables this can be a marvellous way of converting them, especially if the recipe has some noodles in it and a little raw honey (see page 75). As explained earlier, only ever stir-fry with extra-virgin olive oil, which is heat-stable (the polyunsaturated oils such as sunflower and safflower are not heat-stable). If you want to add other oils for flavour, such as walnut oil or sesame oil, sprinkle them on at the end of cooking.

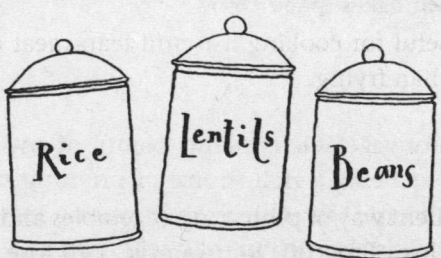

Chapter 6

•

A–Z OF SUPERFOODS FOR THE IMMUNE SYSTEM

Blackcurrants

Very rich in vitamin C, blackcurrants help to strengthen the immune system and are a great source of antioxidants and anthocyanidins (see page 48). You can now buy tinned blackcurrants in juice (as opposed to sugar-laden 'syrup'), which make an excellent ingredient for a smoothie (see page 232).

Blueberries

Rich in anthocyanidins (see page 48), these berries are effective against some forms of *E. coli*. They are also a rich source of vitamin C, and as they are naturally sweet they can be eaten raw or in Blueberry Pancakes (page 167).

Broccoli

This green leafy vegetable contains plenty of antioxidant vitamins, as well as being a rich source of phytonutrients such as chlorophyll and indoles which are powerful anti-cancer compounds. Broccoli is also rich in folic acid, iron and potassium. It makes an excellent cooked finger food for babies or can be steamed or stir-fried for older children.

Brown rice

This is a gluten-free grain, rich in a variety of nutrients including calcium, magnesium, iron, phosphorus, zinc, vitamin E and vitamins B3, B5 and B6. These are all required for a healthy immune system. Brown rice is also an excellent source of fibre, helping to keep your child's digestive tract healthy. As it is gluten-free, it makes an excellent weaning food. You can buy many different varieties: long grain, short grain and sweet brown rice which makes delicious rice puddings. Rice milk is an excellent traditional remedy for infant diarrhoea. It is also very useful as a substitute to cow's milk when your children are ill – unlike dairy products, it is not mucous-forming.

Cinnamon

One of the wonder culinary spices for the immune system, cinnamon has both antibacterial and antifungal properties. It is a perfect winter warmer and makes a lovely addition to puddings and Middle Eastern foods. It warms the whole system and acts as a tonic, combating weakness during viral infections such as flu. Make a warming toddy for your child by filling a mug with hot water and 2 teaspoons tea tree honey (Manuka), the juice of a lemon and quarter of a cinnamon stick. Allow to steep for ten minutes, then remove the cinnamon stick and give the warm toddy to your child.

Cloves

This spice has traditionally been used for toothache, as cloves are antimicrobial and have a powerful antiseptic effect. They are also warming and form a delicious addition to puddings such as apple crumble and some mild curries such as Chickpea and Coconut Curry (page 181).

Extra-virgin olive oil

Olive oil is rich in antioxidant nutrients, especially vitamin E, as well as plenty of phyto-nutrients with antioxidant properties. Always choose the cold-pressed kind. It is a rich dark green and, although more expensive, tastes delicious and retains all its antioxidant properties. Olive oil is an excellent fat for cooking at high temperatures, for example, stir-frying, as it is heat-stable.

Flaxseed oil

A marvellous source of omega-3 essential fatty acids, this oil should be kept in the fridge at all times. It can be added to cooked food, mixed into smoothies or made into dressings (Salad Dressing 2, page 217).

Game

Becoming more popular today, wild game is a fantastic food for the immune system. It is much lower in saturated fat than lamb or beef and is rich in the iron that is so necessary for growing children. Organic game is free-range and therefore free of the antibiotics and hormones regularly fed to intensively farmed animals. If eaten in season, game is also quite cheap. My favourites to cook for the family are venison, wild duck and pheasant. Good sources of free-range and organic game are in the Resources at the back of this book.

Garlic

The king of superfoods for the immune system, garlic has anti-bacterial, antiviral and antifungal properties. It thins the blood, keeping the cardiovascular system healthy. The active components are the phytonutrient allicin and other sulphur-bearing substances. These are the smelly bits! Garlic is a wonderful food to include in your family's diet from a young age. Add it raw to a salad dressing (page 217) or use it to make Hummus (page 148). If you are using it to combat infection it must be used raw, so add some at the end of cooking time.

Ginger

Another warming, antiseptic spice, ginger can be added to stir-fries and curries or used in a hot toddy to combat colds or infections. See also Immune-boosting Soup, page 250.

Herbs

Buy and use fresh wherever possible, or grow your own in pots or a window-box. See also Oregano, Parsley and Thyme.

Juices

Raw fruit and vegetable juices are full of antioxidants and plant enzymes, a package of vitality that will strengthen your child's immune system and provide a naturally sweet and health-promoting alternative to soft drinks. Fresh apple juice, carrot and apple, and lime and pineapple are some good examples. Having a good juicer (see page 64) is a great help. In my family the children do their own juicing, deciding what mixtures to try out and which to throw out! It is just like cooking to them – they are involved, and they get an immediate reward for their efforts. Frozen bananas in a Champion juicer make the most delicious totally natural banana ice cream (see page 153).

Nuts

Packed full of nutrients, nuts are an excellent source of protein, fat, calcium and iron for vegans and vegetarians. They are a good alternative to dairy products and can be mixed with water and blended to create nut milks and creams. My favourite nuts to feed a family are almonds, cashews and walnuts (see Quick Nut Burgers, page 206, and Walnut Cookies, page 157).

Oily fish

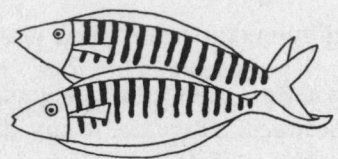

- Salmon

- Mackerel

- Herrings

These are all oily fish rich in omega-3 fatty acids, vital for your child's immune system (see Fish Kebabs, page 178). Wherever possible choose an unpolluted and unfarmed source, as oily fish does retain harmful residues of pollutants (see Resources).

Oregano

Very much a winter herb, oregano has antibacterial properties and helps relieve chest infections, coughs and catarrh. Sprinkle over Colourful Chips (page 141) before cooking, or add to soups and stews.

Parsley

This is my all-time favourite superfood for the immune system. Rich in antioxidant vitamins A and C, as well as chlorophyll, iron, magnesium and other trace elements, it is a must for every fridge, back garden or window-box.

Raw foods

Here we see nutrition at its best. The fresher the better, and the higher the nutrient content will be. Rich in antioxidants and phytonutrients, raw food helps to build a healthy immune system. Cooking destroys nutrients, and there is nothing that will put children off vegetables faster than school dinners with soggy, overcooked veg. Introduce raw fruit and vegetables to your children as babies, and they will grow up loving them.

Seaweed

A wealth of natural trace minerals, vitamins and amino acids are found in seaweed. There are many different types, the most popular being nori, which is wrapped around rice in Japanese sushi. The easiest way to introduce seaweeds to your family is to crumble a little nori into soups or mix it with mashed potato. Alternatively you can use the powdered seaweeds, which can be sprinkled on food. Only use a little at a time, as they do taste quite strong (see Resources).

Seeds

These are little powerhouses of nutrition, for each seed contains all that is needed to grow life.

Dull grey sunflower seeds can turn into beautiful bright yellow flowers, and small green pumpkin seeds can transform into huge orange pumpkins. Here are the seeds that I use in this book:

- **Sesame seeds and sesame seed paste (tahini):** Rich source of omega-6 essential fatty acids, protein, calcium, magnesium, zinc, and vitamins B3 and E. Tahini can be added to a baby's vegetable purée or used in hummus or as a nutty spread.

- **Sunflower seeds:** Wonderful flavour, and a good source of omega-6 fats, protein and B vitamins. They make a great snack food and are lovely sprinkled on a salad or included in baking (see Muesli Bars, page 136).

- **Pumpkin seeds:** Contain the highest level of zinc of all the seeds, as well as notable amounts of iron and calcium. A good source of omega-6 and omega-3 essential fatty acids.

- **Flaxseeds/linseeds:** Wonderful source of fibre and omega-3 essential fatty acids. For older children, grind them in a coffee grinder and add them to cereals. The oil is a concentrated source of omega-3 oils and is easy to disguise in children's food.

Shiitake mushrooms

These oriental mushrooms are super immune-boosters. They possess antibacterial, antiviral and antiparasitic properties and are a natural source of interferon, which provides protection against viruses. They are also a good source of germanium, an element that enhances immunity. Shiitake mushrooms are great in stews, soups or stir-fries (see Immune-boosting Venison, page 228).

Sprouted seeds, pulses, nuts and grains

These little sprouts are cheap, easy to produce and packed with immune-boosting nutrients. Children love to make them and watch them grow. As a raw food, they can be added to salads and popped into pittas or wholemeal sandwiches to boost the nutritional content.

All you need to do is take a handful of seeds, pulses or grains and place them in a bowl. Pick over the seeds and remove any broken ones or bits of dirt. Rinse them well and then soak overnight in tepid water for up to twelve hours. Then drain them, rinse them and put them in a jam jar. Rinse them twice a day in a colander. Drain them well and try not to shake them about too much. Depending on what you are sprouting, they will be ready in two to six days. Put them in a closable polythene bag in the fridge and they will last up to a week.

The easiest ones to start with are alfalfa, aduki, chickpea and mung. You can then progress to barley and wheat grains, sesame, sunflower and pumpkin seeds.

Sugar substitutes

- **Fruit juice concentrates**. These are an excellent alternative to sugary drinks or squashes that contain sugar, colouring and artificial sweeteners. They are very strong and therefore need to be diluted 1/10 with water. They can be frozen into thirst-quenching lollies in the summer or added to smoothies for additional flavour. Apple and blackcurrant is the favourite in our family.

- **Barley malt syrup**. This thick, toffee-like syrup is derived from barley sprouts and water. Rich in maltose, it has a mild taste and is only 40 per cent as sweet as sugar, supplying a more prolonged source of energy than most concentrated sweeteners. It is an excellent alternative to sugar in baking (see Flapjacks, page 184). It can also be enjoyed with Mini Raisin Scotch Pancakes (see page 155).

- **Fructose**. You can buy packs of fructose in most supermarkets. It is fruit sugar and can be used in place of refined white sugar. It is very sweet and is not my first choice of sweeteners (though you do need less), but can be very useful in baking when consistency is important and other sugar substitutes won't do.

- **Raw honey**. Honey that is raw, unfiltered, unheated and unpolluted is antibacterial and an excellent alternative to sugar as it is health-promoting. It contains vitamins, enzymes and minerals which are all utilised by the body as a food. Generally, the darker the honey the richer in minerals it is. This honey comes in runny or thick versions and is quite the most delicious that I have ever tasted. It is great in dressings and stir-fries as well as baking (see Honey Cakes, page 185). Do not give honey to babies under one year old as there is a risk of infection. Honey can contain spores of Clostridium botulinum and this has been a rare, but dangerous, source of infection for infants.

- **Tea tree honey (Manuka).** A real superfood, this honey contains antibacterial and anti-viral properties. It is excellent for soothing sore throats and chasing bugs away. Put two teaspoons of tea tree honey into a mug with the juice of a lemon and fill it with hot (not boiling) water. Allow it to cool slightly before giving it to your child. It has a strong flavour and therefore it is best suited for spreading or using medicinally. Do not give honey to babies under one year old as there is a risk of infection (see above).

- **Molasses.** This superb substance is a by-product of sugar refining – the bit that contains all the minerals stripped out of the sugar. It is an especially good source of calcium and iron, and therefore an excellent addition to your child's diet. It can be given to a baby at six months (see Apple and Molasses Purée, page 94), or added to puddings such as Baked Fruit and Proper Custard (page 230), or used to sweeten puddings or cereals. It has an extremely strong taste, so only add a very little at a time, especially on to cereals (see Protein-packed Porridge, page 137).

- **Maize malt syrup.** This is identical to barley malt syrup except that it is made from corn (maize). It is lighter in colour than the barley version and therefore may suit flour-based cakes and biscuits. It is low in glucose and high in maltose, and therefore releases more sustainable energy.

• **Maple syrup**. Another useful sugar substitute, maple syrup should be used in small amounts as it is very sweet and has a strong flavour which not everyone likes.

Thyme

With its antiviral and antibacterial properties thyme is a great tonic for the body's natural immunity. It is a very useful herb to use when there are coughs and colds around.

Immune makers and breakers

Immune makers

• Fresh organic vegetables, raw, steamed, stir-fried or juiced to retain nutrients
• Fresh organic fruit, raw, baked or juiced to retain nutrients
• Wholegrains such as wholemeal bread and pasta, oats, brown rice, millet and quinoa made into cereals, as an accompaniment, or in soups and stews
• Nuts and seeds
• Poultry and game
• Organic eggs
• Organic cheese and yoghurt (as long as the eater has no allergies)
• Fresh fish, especially oily ones (e.g. salmon, herrings, mackerel, tuna, pilchards, anchovies) from unpolluted sources
• Pulses and beans (e.g. lentils, chickpeas, flageolet, haricot, kidney and butter beans)
• Organic soya products (e.g. soya milk, yoghurt, tofu, tempeh)
• Unhydrogenated margarines or a little butter for spreading

continues ▶

- Extra-virgin olive oil for cooking and dressings
- Flaxseed oil or an oil blend (see Resources), added to food, in dressings or in shakes

Immune breakers

- White bread and pasta
- White flour and cakes and biscuits made from it
- Tinned fruit in syrup
- Jellies (except home-made from fresh juice) and packet puddings
- Jams and marmalades (except 100 per cent fruit jams)
- Packet and tinned soups
- Chips (except home-made baked chips)
- Crisps
- Fizzy drinks which contain sugar, colouring and artificial sweeteners
- Cream and ice cream (except home-made)
- Margarines and processed golden cooking oils
- Caffeine, found in coffee, tea, chocolate, chocolate drinks and some fizzy drinks
- Salt

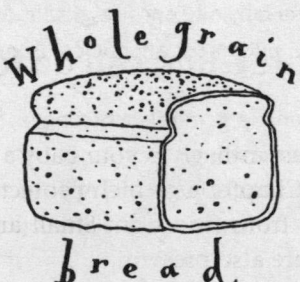

Chapter 7

•

BABY IMMUNE POWER — THE FIRST SIX MONTHS

As soon as your baby is born, her immune system starts functioning. However, it is immature. It has not yet encountered the many thousands of different germs, viruses, fungi and bacteria that she will be exposed to through her life. Her lymphocytes are also not able to make all the different antibodies that she will need. This happens slowly through the first year of her life. During this period, breast-feeding your baby is the best possible support that you can give her immune system. It will protect her against allergies and against infections more common in bottle-fed babies, as well as supplying her with substances that actively help her immune system develop.

What breast-feeding can do for your baby

- **Antibodies.** Breast milk gives your baby a good supply of IgA antibodies (see Chapter 1) which protect her intestinal and respiratory tract from infection. Small amounts of IgG and IgM antibodies are also present.

- **Antioxidants.** Breast milk, especially colostrum, which is produced in the first three days before the milk comes in, is rich in protein and minerals as well as vitamins A and E and B12. There is far more selenium, a powerful antioxidant, in breast milk than in formula milks.

● **Minerals**. Zinc in breast milk is more easily absorbed than zinc in formula milks. This mineral is essential for the development of the thymus gland, which plays a key role in your baby's immune system development. Iron in breast milk, too, is more easily absorbed than in formula milks. Lactoferrin, an iron-binding protein (basically, it renders the iron easier to absorb) is also present in breast milk. In addition lactoferrin inhibits the growth of bacteria, which protects your baby against infection.

● **Enzymes**. Breast milk contains milk-digesting enzymes which break down the fat in milk to form free fatty acids, which inhibit the growth of parasites in your baby's intestines. They are especially effective at killing Giardia, a parasite that can cause diarrhoea in babies.

● **Essential fatty acids**. Breast milk supplies plenty of the EFAs required for the production of prostaglandins, which in turn regulate the activity of the cells of the immune system. These EFAs help to protect your baby from allergies. Formula milk does contain EFAs, but only in small quantities.

● **Anti-microbial factors:**
  • Lysozyme: an antibacterial enzyme that breaks down bacterial cell walls. The lysozyme content of breast milk is 3,000 times higher than that of cow's milk
  • Complement: assists in bacterial cell breakdown
  • Anti-staphylococcal factor: breast milk contains a fat with anti-staphylococcal action
  • Bifidus factor: the presence of Bifidus promotes the growth of beneficial bacteria and provides an acid environment which suppresses bacteria growth.

During these first six months I recommend breast-feeding exclusively, especially if allergies run in the family, as this will help to protect your baby. Between six months and a year I recommend that you breast-feed morning and night, which will protect your baby's maturing immune system.

Healthy mothers, healthy babies

It is important to look after yourself when you are breast-feeding. Your baby effectively eats what you are eating, so here are some helpful hints to ensure that you both keep well.

- Eat five portions of fruit and vegetables a day. This will supply you both with plenty of antioxidants and phytonutrients.

- Have freshly made vegetable and fruit juices in the morning as a vitamin tonic.

- Take a daily supplement of EFAs such as Essential Balance (see Resources).

- Don't skip meals, which will make you more tired and diminish your milk supply.

- Drink plenty of purified water. Breast-feeding makes you very thirsty and your body needs more to produce the milk.

- Snack on fruit and seeds and healthy bars and biscuits, not on chocolate bars and cakes. This will supply valuable vitamins and minerals rather than empty calories.

- Eat when you are hungry and have plenty of healthy snacks around. Breast-feeding increases your appetite.

Immune-boosting recipes for breast-feeding mums

While you are breast-feeding you will need to eat foods that are rich in iron, zinc, calcium and essential fatty acids. Here is a list of recipes rich in these nutrients.

- Liquid Energy Breakfast (omitting the raw egg yolk; page 196)

- Nut and Seed Bread (page 229)

- Panna (page 211)

- Quick and Easy Chicken Liver Pâté (page 200)

- The Very Best Immune-boosting Soup for All the Family (page 249)

- Red Lentil and Spinach Lasagne (page 146)

- Family Fish Pie (page 150)

- Fresh Tuna and Sesame Balls (page 180)

- Immune-boosting Venison (page 228)

- Pumpkin Seed Porridge (page 198)

- Bouillabaisse (page 214)

- Roasted Nut and Vegetable Couscous (page 172)

- Muesli Bars (page 136)

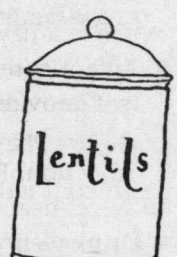

What about bottle-feeding?

To boost your baby's immune system, breast-feeding is unbeatable. However, there are obviously times when breast-feeding is not an option – for example, when you are taking certain drugs or have had breast surgery. For women who have no choice, here are my guidelines.

Making the best of the bottle

- To ensure adequate intake of omega-3 essential fatty acids, add a few drops of flaxseed oil into each bottle after warming. You can now get Dri-celle flaxseed oil which mixes better with formula. Give your baby a maximum of one teaspoon of oil in a twenty-four-hour period. If it is hard to remember, you can add a whole teaspoon of oil to a bottle once a day.

- To ensure adequate intake of omega-6 essential fatty acids, rub the contents of an Efamol Evening Primrose Oil capsule on to your baby's tummy once a day.

- Once a day, add a quarter of a teaspoon of Bifidobacterium Infantis (see Resources) to the milk just before feeding. This will provide your baby with the beneficial bacteria she would get in breast milk and help to protect her from intestinal infection. Keep the Bifidobacteria Infantis in the fridge and never heat it, or you will kill it.

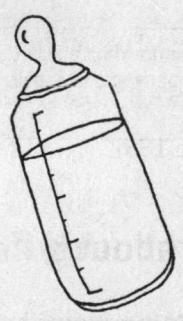

Chapter 8

•

BABY IMMUNE POWER – SIX TO NINE MONTHS

Nutrient focus chart

Nutrient	Function	Source
Iron	Prevents anaemia and helps the body to resist infection	Dried fruit, spring greens, spinach, parsley, poultry, chicken liver, red lentils, lamb, wholegrain rice
Beta-carotene	Vegetable source of vitamin A; strengthens mucous membranes as first line of defence	Butternut squash, pumpkin, cantaloupe melon, carrots, sweet potatoes, apricots, green leafy vegetables
Vitamin C	Powerful antioxidant which is both antibacterial and antiviral	Broccoli, parsley, kiwi fruit, blackcurrants, Brussels sprouts, papaya, mangoes

Introducing first foods

At around the age of six months your baby will be ready for solid food. At this time, her immune system will start to hold its own. She will continue to develop her ability to produce different antibodies right the way through her first year of life. Delaying weaning until she is six months old will have reduced the risk of her developing allergies, especially if problems such as asthma, eczema, migraine or hay fever run in the family.

Baby foods – the golden rules

In order to build on the strength of your baby's immunity there are some golden rules that I have put together for introducing these first foods.

1. Avoid foods that are likely to cause an allergic reaction. Eighty per cent of such reactions are caused by just eight foods:

- peanuts
- tree nuts (pecans, walnuts etc.)
- fish
- shellfish
- eggs
- milk
- soya
- wheat

None of these foods should be introduced as first foods.

2. Use fresh foods whenever you can – the fresher the better. These contain more of the vitamins and minerals that are essential for your baby's immune system. Long storage times deplete the food of its nutrient content.

3. Use wholegrains instead of refined baby grains (e.g. baby rice, baby pasta), because they have a greater range of nutrients. Suitable grains at this age are rice, millet, quinoa and buckwheat. Recent research has indicated that up to a third of heart diseases and cancers could be prevented simply by eating three daily portions of wholegrains. Initiating this routine at an early age will ensure that your baby is on the road to good health and not to disease.

4. To avoid allergies, make purées of single fruit and vegetables and introduce them one at a time, then repeat them over two or three days so that your baby gets used to them. This makes it easy to see if she is reacting to a particular food. After that you can start creating different combinations (see Menu Planner at the end of the chapter).

5. Slowly introduce a wide variety of different foods so that your baby develops an adventurous appetite. This will also ensure that she gets a broad selection of the nutrients needed for optimal immune function.

6. During the weaning process give your baby as much organic produce as possible. At this age babies eat far more fruit, vegetables and grains, weight for weight, than adults do. They are therefore at a much higher risk of consuming unsafe levels of pesticides, some of which are known to be carcinogenic. Your baby will be exposed to plenty of chemicals and pollutants in her early life, so reducing her immune burden whenever possible is a bonus. If you were only to feed your children organic food once in their lives, this would be the best time.

Helpful hint

You don't need a load of expensive kit for feeding your baby her first food. All you need to buy is some plastic baby spoons. Rather than buying weaning bowls you can use the tops of feeding bottles, which can be easily sterilised. Alternatively you can use small Tupperware pots, which are also useful when freezing individual pasta sauce portions for older babies. Prepare your baby foods using the ice cube method (see page 65). Start by offering small tastes and gradually increase the amount according to your baby's preferences.

7. Avoid genetically modified foods wherever possible. There is a huge debate about the effects of GM foods on the environment and on our health. Choosing organic foods will minimise your child's exposure to GM foods.

8. Up to the age of one, your baby still needs to receive 600 ml (1 pint) of formula or breast milk a day.

Six to nine months

Foods to include	Foods to avoid
Fresh fruit purées	Citrus fruit and strawberries*
Fresh vegetable purées	Potato, tomato, aubergine, peppers (see note)
Dried fruit purées	Eggs*
Gluten-free grain purées including rice, millet, buckwheat, quinoa	Gluten grains (wheat*, barley, rye and oats)
Pulses and bean purées	Dairy products⁴ (milk, yoghurt, cream, cheese)
Organic poultry, game and meat purées	Nuts and seeds*
Fish purées* (except shellfish)	Soya products* (soya milk, tofu, tempeh, TVP)
	Corn*
	Honey (see note)
	Shellfish*

The foods marked with an asterisk are the ones most likely to cause an allergic reaction of some kind and therefore their introduction is delayed.

Potatoes, tomatoes, aubergines and red, yellow and green peppers belong to the deadly nightshade family and can provoke symptoms. They are better introduced at nine months rather than six.

Honey is not given to babies under one year old because it can contain spores of *Clostridium botulinum* (see page 62) that can cause food poisoning.

Commercial baby foods

When you are shopping for baby foods, whether jars or dried, here are some helpful hints to prevent your being misled by the manufacturers.

- **Don't buy jars, rusks or cereal-based baby foods that contain wheat**, even if the packet or jar says 'suitable from four months'. The government has produced guidelines saying that no gluten should be introduced until six months, because of the risk of developing coeliac disease. Some baby food manufacturers are choosing to ignore these guidelines.

- **Check the labels for sugar**. Any baby food sweetened with added sugar is totally unacceptable. Sugar suppresses your baby's immune system. Don't be fooled by low-sugar varieties of baby foods. One popular brand of rusk which claims to be 'reduced sugar' still has 21 per cent sugar – even more than in a jam doughnut (19 per cent)! If you want teething rusks, give your baby rice cakes, peeled apple slices or big carrot sticks (don't give her anything that she might choke on).

- **Look out for hidden ingredients**. What comes first on the ingredients list is the largest component by percentage. If it is soya formula, the largest component will be glucose syrup (i.e. sugar). If the first ingredient listed on a jar of baby food is water, don't buy it – for obvious reasons it is bad value. Some brands clearly state that they don't add starches, while others contain more than the ingredients mentioned in the name of the product. For example, Cow and Gate Sage and Turkey Casserole contains more maltodextrin than turkey, and Sainsbury's Sunshine Banana has more maltodextrin and sugar than banana.

- **Watch out for misleading labels**. Sainsbury's Five Fruits Yoghurt contains more sugar than fruit, and Cow and Gate Banana Rice contains no banana, just banana flavouring.

- **The best of the brands**. The Which? report May 2000 revealed that the only brand of baby food, both jar and dried, that does not use sugar or starches in its meals is Baby Organix.

- **The best solution** is to make your own organic baby food and keep a few fruit jars for puddings and travelling.

Recipes

Making fresh fruit and vegetable purées is the best introduction to food that you can offer your baby. They are very quick to prepare and you don't need lots of equipment. Steaming is the best cooking method, as it retains more nutrients than boiling. Vitamins B and C are water-soluble. This means that they are leached into the cooking water when you boil vegetables, and therefore unless you use all the cooking water you lose a lot of the nutrients. If you don't have a steamer you can use a colander over a pan and put a lid on top.

Remember to make the first purées very runny so that your baby, being used only to liquids, enjoys her first food sensation. Below is an example of a single-ingredient purée. Once your baby has tried out single purées, you will find you can quickly move on to double and triple fruit and vegetable purées (see menu on pages 108). I have indicated how many ice cubes these first purées will make, but this is only a guide as the quantity made will obviously depend on the size of both the ice cube trays and the vegetables.

Key ro recipes

(V) = vegetarian   [df] = dairy-free

(V) = vegan   [gf] = gluten-free

[wf] = wheat-free   * = can be frozen

Butternut Squash Purée*

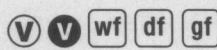

Butternut squash makes a lovely, smooth, sweet purée that all babies love. It is also rich in beta-carotene, which is a super immune-boosting vitamin.

MAKES ABOUT 18 CUBES

1 butternut squash
filtered water for steaming

Peel, deseed and chop the squash. Steam for 10 minutes until very soft. Purée to the desired consistency, using some of the steamed vegetable water if necessary.

Other excellent single purées for a healthy immune system

Apple, apricot, beetroot, broccoli, cantaloupe melon, carrot, dried fruit, green cabbage, kale, kiwi fruit, mango, nectarine, papaya, parsnip, peach, plum, pumpkin, spinach, swede, sweet potato

---

Pumpkin and Parsley Purée*

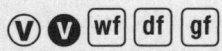

This purée is packed with immune-boosting nutrients. The pumpkin is a good source of beta-carotene and vitamin E, while the parsley adds vitamin C and iron in useful amounts. Babies love this purée for its sweetness, and it is exceptionally good for them as well!

MAKES ABOUT 20 CUBES

1 pumpkin
a handful parsley
filtered water for steaming

Peel, deseed and chop the pumpkin. Chop the parsley and steam together with the pumpkin for 10–15 minutes, until soft. Purée to the desired consistency, using some of the steamed vegetable water if necessary.

Broccoli and Sweet Potato Purée*

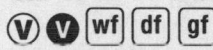

Another magic combination that babies love. Broccoli is a real superfood for the immune system. It is rich in carotenoids, iron, folic acid and vitamin C. Sweet potatoes are not related to ordinary potatoes, despite the name, and are unlikely to cause an allergic reaction. This makes them an ideal weaning food.

MAKES ABOUT 24 CUBES

1 head organic broccoli
4 sweet potatoes (organic if available)
filtered water for steaming

Remove the heavy stalk and chop the broccoli into florets. Peel and chop the sweet potatoes and steam both vegetables together for 10–15 minutes, until soft. Purée to the desired consistency.

Blueberry and Apple Purée*

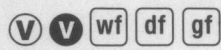

Blueberries contain antibacterial compounds called anthocyanidins, which are particularly effective against some forms of *E. coli* bacteria, the main culprits in tummy upsets. You can now buy jars of organic apple and blueberry purée, which are great to use when travelling or going out.

MAKES ABOUT 20 CUBES

1 kg (just over 2 lb) bag organic eating apples
1 punnet organic blueberries
filtered water for steaming

Peel, core and chop the apples. Wash the blueberries well. Steam the fruit together for 10–12 minutes until nice and soft, then purée to the desired consistency.

Kiwi, Mango and Banana Purée

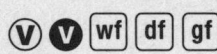

Kiwi fruit contain more vitamin C than oranges and as much vitamin E as an avocado. Mangoes are packed full of beta-carotene, which helps to strengthen the immune system. Combined with banana, this makes a lovely smooth purée ideal for warding off colds.

MAKES 1 SERVING

1 kiwi fruit
½ very ripe mango
1 small banana or ½ big banana

Scoop out the kiwi fruit flesh and peel the mango, then remove the mango flesh from the large stone. Peel the banana and purée all the fruit together to the desired consistency.

Banana and Nectarine Purée

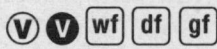

Another delicious summer combination, full of vitamin C for a healthy immune system.

MAKES 1 SERVING

½ ripe nectarine
1 small banana or ½ large banana

Halve, stone and peel the nectarine, then purée with the banana to the desired consistency.

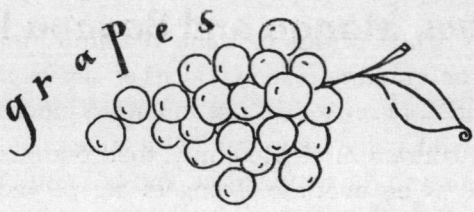

Apple and Molasses Purée*

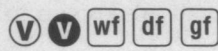

The molasses in this recipe adds useful amounts of iron and calcium.

MAKES ABOUT 24 CUBES

1 kg (just over 2 lb) bag organic eating apples
filtered water for steaming
1 level teaspoon blackstrap molasses

Peel, core and slice the apples, then steam until soft. Drizzle in the molasses and purée to the desired consistency.

Spinach and Parsnip Purée*

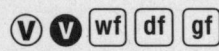

Spinach is rich in carotenoids and vitamin C, important nutrients for the immune system. However, although spinach is a useful source of iron, it does not contain as much as Popeye portrayed! A food analyst who was doing some calculations put the decimal point in the wrong place, and as a result it was believed for a long time that spinach had ten times more iron than it did! Spinach also has a very strong taste due to the oxalic acid it contains, which inhibits the absorption of calcium and iron. But if you combine spinach with a vegetable or fruit containing vitamin C, such as parsnip, the iron within it is more easily absorbed (and it also tastes much better). And combining it with this or another root vegetable, such as swede, turnip, sweet potato, carrot or celeriac, makes a nice smooth purée. Do try to find organic spinach, as a report published in *Reader's Digest* in 1996 showed an alarming one in three spinach leaves sampled in the UK exceed the safe limit of nitrates, which are known to be carcinogenic.

MAKES ABOUT 15 CUBES

4 large organic parsnips
1 bag organic baby leaf spinach
filtered water for steaming

Peel and chop the parsnip, wash the spinach and steam together for 10 minutes until soft. Purée to the desired consistency. Spinach retains a lot of water, so you are unlikely to need to add any extra.

> **Helpful hint**
> Other useful alternatives to spinach are kale, spring greens and watercress.

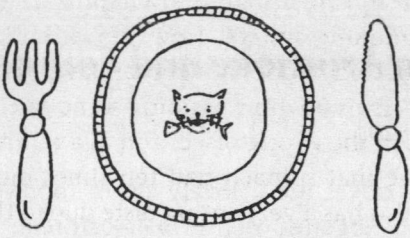

Celeriac and Cauliflower Purée*

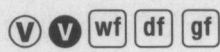

Celeriac is another winter root vegetable which makes a nice base for a vegetable purée. It contains vitamin C, which is important for keeping your baby's immune system strong. Cauliflower is part of the cruciferous family of vegetables, which includes broccoli and all forms of cabbage. Cruciferous vegetables contain compounds which offer some protection against cancer.

MAKES ABOUT 20 CUBES

1 organic celeriac
1 small organic cauliflower
filtered water for steaming

Peel and chop the celeriac. Wash the cauliflower and remove the outer leaves. Break into florets and steam the vegetables together for 10–15 minutes until soft. Purée to the desired consistency, using some of the steamed vegetable water if necessary.

Jerusalem Artichoke and Courgette Purée*

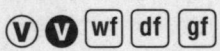

Jerusalem artichokes are a lovely sweet root vegetable which babies enjoy. Courgettes, rich in beta-carotene and vitamin C, are best combined with a root vegetable because, with their high water content, they make a very thin purée on their own. In traditional Chinese medicine Jerusalem artichokes are used for strengthening the lungs, so they are an excellent food to serve to your baby and later on in her childhood when there are chest infections around.

MAKES ABOUT 16 CUBES

5–6 medium Jerusalem artichokes
2 organic courgettes
filtered water for steaming

Peel and chop the artichokes. Wash the courgettes, top and tail them and chop the rest. Steam both vegetables together for 10 minutes until soft, then purée to the desired consistency.

First Cereals

Millet Porridge

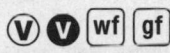

This recipe is taken from my first book, *Optimum Nutrition for Babies and Young Children,* because I think it is the very best first breakfast and all three of my children, as well as many others, adored it as babies. Millet is gluten free and an ideal first grain for babies as it is unlikely to cause allergies. It is also rich in iron, potassium and magnesium, good nutrients for a healthy immune system. If you grind the millet flakes in a coffee grinder before cooking, you make millet flour which produces a much smoother porridge. I usually grind a whole pack of flakes and store the flour in an airtight glass container, to save having to muck about every morning! For older babies you can use the millet flakes straight. Zwicky is a good brand available from healthfood shops.

MAKES 1 SERVING

1 tablespoon ground millet flakes
150 ml (5 fl oz) filtered water, breast milk or formula

Put the millet and liquid in a small pan. Bring to the boil, stirring, and simmer for 5–10 minutes until it thickens and is cooked through. Serve with some fruit purée.

Brown Rice Purée*

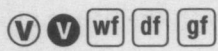

Rice is a gluten-free grain traditionally used as a weaning food. Sweet brown rice (see Resources) makes a creamier, richer purée than ordinary brown rice and babies love it. If you freeze this purée using the ice cube method, you can use a couple of cubes with some fresh fruit purée for an instant meal.

MAKES ABOUT 30 CUBES

1 cup short grain brown rice or sweet brown rice
4 cups filtered water

Put the rice and water in a small pan and bring to the boil, stirring. Gently simmer, covered, for 30–40 minutes until the rice is very soft. Check the water level from time to time – you may need to add more if it's absorbed too quickly.

Banana, Quinoa and Millet porridge

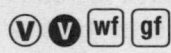

Quinoa is rich in protein, calcium and iron and therefore an excellent food to incorporate in your baby's diet for a healthy immune system. You can buy this grain from healthfood shops or direct from mail order companies (see Resources).

MAKES 1 SERVING

2 teaspoons quinoa flakes
1 dessertspoon millet flakes
150 ml (5 fl oz) filtered water, breast milk or formula
1 small or ½ large banana

Put the quinoa flakes, millet flakes and water in a pan, bring to the boil, stirring, and simmer gently for 30 minutes until the grains are soft. Purée or mash the porridge with the banana to the desired consistency.

First savoury meals

Cod, Broccoli and Sweet Potato*

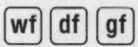 wf df gf

Cod, being a deep-sea fish, is likely to contain fewer pollutants than shallow-water fish such as plaice. Combining the cod with broccoli and sweet potato creates a wonderfully complete meal and supplies all the vitamins, minerals and micronutrients required by a healthy immune system.

MAKES ABOUT 18 CUBES

100 g (4 oz) skinless, boneless cod fillet
1 head organic broccoli
2 large sweet potatoes
filtered water for steaming

Rinse the cod under cold, filtered water. Peel and chop the sweet potato into bite-size pieces and put in the steamer. Wash the broccoli, remove the thick stem, cut the rest into florets and add to the steamer. Steam the vegetables for 20 minutes, adding the fish after 10 minutes, then purée to the desired consistency.

Wild Salmon Pasta*

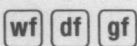 wf df gf

Wild salmon is the most delicious of fish. It has a natural pink colour in contrast to farmed salmon, which tends to look artificially pink and is pumped full of antibiotics and hormones. Rice pasta has the advantage of being gluten-free and is therefore perfect for this age group. If you cannot find rice pasta, use brown rice flakes, which are available from healthfood shops.

MAKES ABOUT 14 CUBES

1 handful rice pasta
1 spring onion, washed and finely sliced
1 tablespoon extra-virgin olive oil
1 skinless, boneless wild salmon fillet, cubed
1 handful organic baby leaf spinach, washed

Cook the rice pasta in boiling water for 10–15 minutes until soft. While it is cooking, gently sauté the spring onion in a pan with the olive oil for 3–4 minutes. Add the cubes of salmon fillet to the pan and sauté for 5–6 minutes until cooked. Toss in the spinach and sauté for another 2–3 minutes until it shrivels. Drain the pasta and add to the salmon pan. Stir the mixture together well and purée to the desired consistency.

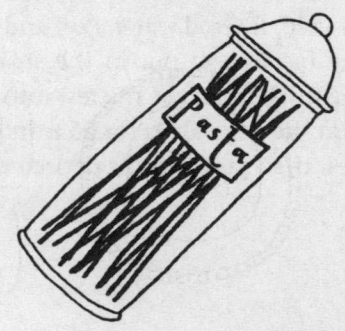

Chicken and Apricots*

wf df gf

Apricots, whether dried or fresh, contain immune-boosting vitamins vital to a healthy immune system. Chicken, with its low allergen potential, is a perfect first savoury food for babies.

MAKES ABOUT 10 CUBES

8 unsulphured dried apricots or 6 fresh organic apricots
  (depending on season)
1 organic skinless, boneless chicken breast
4 tablespoons filtered water
extra-virgin olive oil

If using dried apricots, soak overnight and drain the soaking liquid before using. Preheat the oven to 180°C/350°F/gas 4. Put the chicken breast in a well-oiled ovenproof dish. If using fresh apricots, wash, peel, halve and remove the stones. Surround the chicken with the apricots. Add the water and bake for 20–25 minutes until the chicken is cooked through. Purée all the ingredients together and thin with breast milk, formula or filtered water if necessary. Serve with some additional vegetable purées, for example, two green vegetable cubes and one root vegetable cube such as parsnip, swede or celeriac.

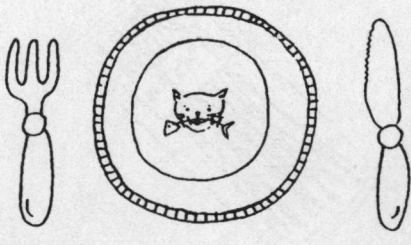

Vegetable Stock*

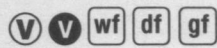

This stock is marvellous to have in the freezer in ice cube portions. It contains thyme, an immune-boosting herb which will stimulate your baby's natural resistance and has both antiviral and antibacterial activity. It also contains garlic – antibacterial, antiviral and antifungal – which has to be the most important item in the immune-boosting larder. It gives added flavour to these very first savoury purées.

MAKES ABOUT 28 CUBES

2 tablespoons extra-virgin olive oil
1 medium onion, peeled and chopped
1 small clove garlic, peeled and crushed
2 large organic carrots, washed, peeled and sliced
3 stalks organic celery including tops, washed and sliced
1 sprig fresh thyme
1 bay leaf
850 ml (1½ pints) filtered water

In a pan, heat the oil and cook the onion and garlic for a few minutes until soft. Add the carrot and celery, stir and cook gently for 5 minutes. Add the thyme, bay leaf and water, bring to the boil, cover and simmer for 1 hour. Remove the bay leaf and thyme before liquidising.

First Chicken and Vegetables*

wf df gf

Most babies love the taste of chicken as it is very mild.

MAKES ABOUT 14 CUBES

1 small leek, washed and sliced
1 tablespoon extra-virgin olive oil
1 organic skinless, boneless chicken breast, cubed
1 organic celery stick, washed and sliced
1 large organic carrot, washed, peeled and sliced
6 cubes frozen vegetable stock (see page 81)

Gently cook the leek in the olive oil in a pan for 5 minutes until soft. Add the chicken cubes and sauté for 5 minutes until white all over. Add the celery and carrot to the pan along with the vegetable stock and simmer for 15 minutes until the chicken is cooked through. Purée to the desired consistency.

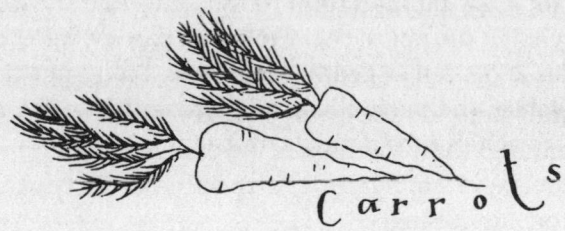

carrots

First Lamb Stew*

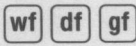 wf df gf

This unseasoned lamb dish has plenty of flavour and is well diluted with vegetables so that it is not too heavy on your baby's digestive system.

MAKES ABOUT 22 CUBES

1 small onion, peeled and finely chopped
1 small clove garlic, peeled and crushed
1 tablespoon extra-virgin olive oil
250 g (8 oz) lamb neck fillet, cubed
½ butternut squash, peeled and cubed
1 organic carrot, washed, peeled and cubed
a handful parsley, washed and chopped
300 ml (½ pint) filtered water *or* fresh vegetable stock
   (see page 102)

Put the onion and garlic in a heavy pan and cook gently in the olive oil for a few minutes until translucent. Add the lamb and brown well. Put the rest of the vegetables, parsley, water or stock in the pan and simmer gently for 1 hour. Scoop out the meat and vegetables and purée them, adding enough of the remaining stock to achieve the desired consistency.

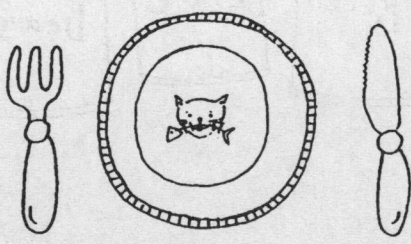

Flageolet Bean Purée*

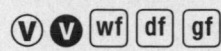

Flageolet beans create a really lovely creamy purée and are packed with the protein required for growth and repair by the immune system. Get a no sugar, no salt variety, available at healthfood shops or from specialist mail order companies (see Resources).

MAKES ABOUT 32 CUBES

1 cup brown rice
filtered water for cooking
1 acorn squash, peeled, deseeded and chopped
1 handful parsley, washed
1 tin cooked flageleot beans

Wash the rice thoroughly, then cook for 35–40 minutes until soft. Meanwhile steam the acorn squash and parsley for 20 minutes until soft. Drain and rinse the beans. Purée all the ingredients together to the desired consistency.

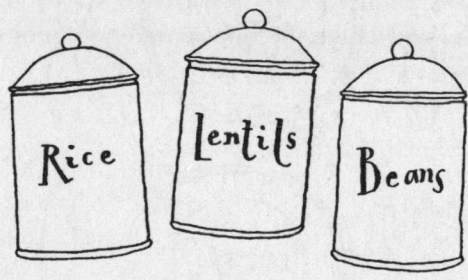

Sprouted Salad Purée

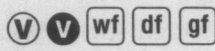

If you can get this purée really smooth, I do not think you will find a more complete baby food. Avocados are rich in the anti-oxidant vitamin E, protein and monounsaturated fat. Sprouted seeds, pulses and grains provide more nutrients ounce for ounce than any other known natural food. You can get them at health-food shops, or else sprout your own (see page 59).

MAKES 1 SERVING

1 tablespoon mixed sprouts
½ small avocado

Liquidise the sprouts to a fine paste, then purée with the avocado and serve immediately.

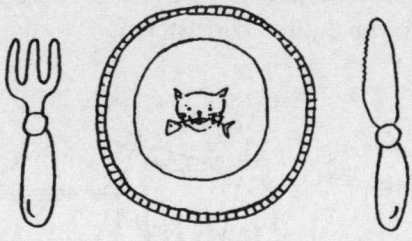

Menu planning and the weaning process

On the following page is a four-week plan which shows you how to introduce food to your baby and how to build up the amount that she is having. As you can see, I have suggested introducing food for the first time at lunchtime. Start off with a milk feed and then in the middle of the feed offer small tastes of purée. Don't worry if your baby fusses at the spoon – it is a new experience for her, and it may take a little while to get used to the sensation. Build up the amounts that you offer, according to your baby's appetite. Once feeding is established some babies will only eat a couple of cubes at each meal, while others will be eating four to six cubes. By seven months your baby will be on three meals a day and, as you introduce more filling purées, you will notice that she starts to drink less milk. If you are breast-feeding she will feed for a shorter time and be less interested than before. Introduce a beaker cup of water at around six months, although most babies don't get the hang of them until eight to ten months. See the chart on pages 108–109.

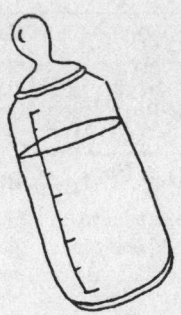

A Four-week weaning plan

WEEK 1	Monday	Tuesday	Wednesday
Breakfast			
Lunch (up to 1 cube in the middle of the milk feed)	Butternut Squash Purée (page 71)	Butternut Squash Purée (page 71)	Carrot purée
Tea			

WEEK 2	Monday	Tuesday	Wednesday
Breakfast			
Lunch (up to 1–2 cubes in the middle of the milk feed)	Banana purée	Sweet potato purée	Sweet potato purée
Tea			

WEEK 3	Monday	Tuesday	Wednesday
Breakfast (up to 2 cubes in the middle of the milk feed)	Millet Porridge (page 97) and pear purée	Millet Porridge (page 97) and pear purée	Brown Rice Purée (page 98) and apple purée
Lunch (2–3 cubes before the milk feed)	Blueberry and Apple Purée (page 92)	Blueberry and Apple Purée (page 92)	Avocado and banana purée
Tea			

WEEK 4	Monday	Tuesday	Wednesday
Breakfast (up to 2–3 cubes in the middle of the milk feed)	Brown Rice Purée (page 98) and pear purée	Millet Porridge (page 97) and apple purée	Brown Rice Purée (page 98) and banana purée
Lunch (up to 2–3 cubes before the milk feed)	Spinach and Parsnip purée (page 94)	Broccoli and Sweet potato purée (page 91)	Carrot and green bean purée
Tea (up to 1–2 cubes before the milk feed)	Avocado and banana purée	Blueberry and Apple Purée (page 92)	Spinach and Parsnip purée (page 94)

Thursday	Friday	Saturday	Sunday
Carrot purée	Apple purée	Apple purée	Banana purée

Thursday	Friday	Saturday	Sunday
Avocado purée	Avocado purée	Pear purée	Pear purée

Thursday	Friday	Saturday	Sunday
Brown Rice Purée (page 98) and apple purée	Millet Porridge (page 97) and banana purée	Millet Porridge (page 97) and banana purée	Brown Rice Purée (page 98) and apple purée
Avocado and banana purée	Pumpkin and Parsley purée (page 90)	Broccoli and Sweet Potato purée (page 91)	Spinach and Parsnip purée (page 94)

Thursday	Friday	Saturday	Sunday
Millet Porridge (page 97) and peach purée	Brown Rice Purée (page 98) and peach purée	Millet Porridge (page 97) and apple purée	Brown Rice Purée (page 98) and pear purée
Butternut Squash purée (page 90)	Banana and Nectarine purée (page 93)	Celeriac and Cauliflower Purée (page 96)	Celeriac and Cauliflower Purée (page 96)
Apple and Molasses purée (page 94)	Broccoli and Sweet Potato purée (page 91)	Pumpkin and Parsley purée (page 90)	Kiwi, Mango and Banana purée (page 92)

Chapter 9

•

BABY IMMUNE POWER – NINE TO TWELVE MONTHS

Nutrient focus chart

Nutrient	Function	Source
Zinc	Needed for the growth and development of white blood cells, part of the immune army	Poultry, game, lean red meat, seeds and nuts, seafood, wholegrains
Essential fatty acids	Help to regulate the activity of the immune system	Flaxseeds, pumpkin seeds, sunflower seeds, salmon, mackerel, fresh tuna, herrings, sardines, walnuts
Magnesium	Required for fatty acid metabolism and antibody production	Wholegrains, pulses, nuts, seeds, dried fruit, green leafy vegetables

Getting more adventurous

At nine months, with a strong immune foundation, your baby can move to an even more adventurous diet as more types of foods can be introduced. As she will be on three meals a day, incorporating meat, fish, grains, vegetables and fruit, she is likely to have dropped her lunchtime and teatime milk feeds and to be drinking water from a feeder cup at these meals. Until she is a year old she still needs to receive 600 ml (1 pint) of breast milk or formula in her diet. Every baby is different, so go with the flow, but by this age my own three children were having a milk feed with breakfast and at bedtime which fulfilled this requirement.

Your baby is likely to have acquired a few teeth by nine months and will have progressed to some well-mashed food instead of a fine purée. Encourage the next stage of eating by offering her some finger foods including:

- baby rice cakes

- peeled, sliced apple pieces

- banana pieces

- ripe pear slices

- steamed carrot sticks

- steamed French beans

- steamed broccoli florets

- fingers of cooked organic chicken

- toasted finger slices of gluten-free bread (such as brown rice bread, available at healthfood shops – these are expensive, but the best available).

Never leave your baby unattended in case of choking.

Babies do like to get involved in feeding themselves at this stage, and you may find that using a splat mat on the floor will minimise the mess! Let your baby use one spoon while you use another. This will keep you both happy and get your baby used to the idea of using implements.

A note about allergies

I have suggested that this is a suitable time to introduce nuts and seeds into your baby's diet. But, as explained earlier, these foods can be highly allergenic, so if there is a history of allergy in the family it would be prudent to delay their introduction until your baby is one year old. I introduced ground nuts and seeds to my own children at nine months as I felt that the health benefits of these foods far outweighed the risks. Introduce the least allergenic first, such as ground almonds and ground sunflower seeds, and progress from there. Important: don't introduce peanut butter until your baby is over a year old, and if there are any close relations with peanut allergy leave it until the child is five. Be aware of the symptoms of an allergic reaction so that you can recognise if your child is sensitive to a particular food:

- vomiting
- itching
- swelling of the lips, throat, tongue, face and head
- rashes
- flushing
- difficulty in breathing

If any of these symptoms occur, don't offer the offending food again for a while. When you do reintroduce it, it is a good idea to be close to your local doctor's surgery or hospital just in case your child reacts severely. The second exposure to an allergen, not the first, is the one that causes the bad reaction.

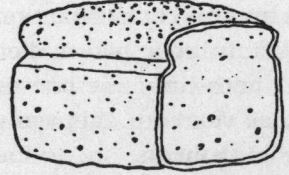

Nine to twelve months

Foods to include	Foods to avoid
Fresh fruit purées	Citrus fruits and strawberries*
Fresh vegetable purées including potato, tomato, aubergine and pepper	
Dried fruit purées	
Grains: oats, barley, rye, corn, rice, millet, buckwheat, quinoa, rice cakes	Wheat*
Organic poultry, game and meat purées	Dairy products*
Fish purées	Shellfish*
Soya products (tofu, soya yoghurt, TVP, tempeh, soya cheese)	Soya milk* (unmodified)
Nuts and seeds: almonds, cashews, sunflower seeds, sesame seeds, pumpkin seeds, seed pastes such as tahini	Peanuts*
Egg yolks	Egg whites*
	Sugar and honey
	Salt

*The foods marked with an asterisk are the ones most likely to cause an allergic reaction of some kind and therefore their introduction is delayed.

Recipes

The recipes in this section concentrate on the foods that you can now introduce into your baby's diet. They also contain foods which are rich in the immune-boosting nutrients featured in the nutrient focus chart for this age group. You will find that many of the recipes in the one-to-four age group are also suitable for your baby at this age if they are mashed or puréed. If you refer to the chart above you can easily double-check this.

All recipes in this chapter serve one baby or are for batch cooking.

Almond and Rice Porridge

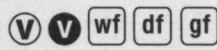

This is one of my favourite breakfasts for this age group.

MAKES 1 SERVING

1 tablespoon ground brown rice flakes
150 ml (5 fl oz) formula, breast milk or water
1 teaspoon organic almond nut butter or 1 teaspoon organic ground almonds
1–2 cubes fruit purée

Put the rice flakes in a pan and cover with the milk or water. Bring to the boil and simmer for 10 minutes until soft. Add the other ingredients, mix, mash and serve.

Alternative porridge mixtures

Instead of the cashews you can grind some almonds or sunflower seeds, pumpkin seeds, sesame seeds or linseeds. You could also add a teaspoon of flaxseed oil to boost the EFA content of the porridge.

Cashew, Dried Apricot and Oat Porridge

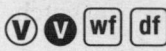

Oats make a wonderful porridge that can be enjoyed by the whole family. They are rich in the B vitamins as well as in magnesium, calcium and potassium. This recipe contains all the components needed to build healthy immune systems.

MAKES 1 SERVING

1 heaped tablespoon porridge oats
filtered water
6 ground cashews
2 cubes Dried Apricot Purée (see opposite)

Put the oats in a pan with enough water to cover. Bring to the boil and simmer for 5 minutes until thickened and cooked through. Once cooked, take off the heat and stir in the ground cashews and dried apricot purée. The porridge will go all creamy and sticky.

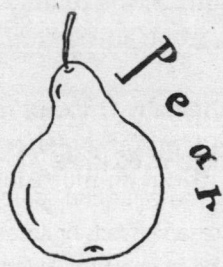

Dried Apricot Purée*

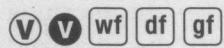

Dried apricots are a delicious addition to grains or fruit purées. They are a great source of beta-carotene. This purée is very sweet, so I suggest you do not give it to your baby as a single purée.

MAKES ABOUT 35 CUBES

450 g (1 lb) packet unsulphured dried apricots
filtered water

Place the apricots in a bowl and cover with filtered water. Soak overnight. In the morning transfer the apricots and water to a pan. Bring to the boil, then simmer gently for 20 minutes until the apricots are nice and soft. Purée to the desired consistency. This purée is quite gluey when frozen, which makes it rather sticky to handle.

Pear, Apple and Oats

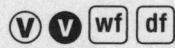

This idea came from the Baby Organix range of baby foods. It is so easy to prepare and makes a perfect breakfast or pudding (though the jars are without doubt easier if you are travelling or out and about).

MAKES 1 SERVING

1 tablespoon oat flakes
1 teaspoon sun-dried raisins
filtered water
1 cube apple purée
1 cube pear purée

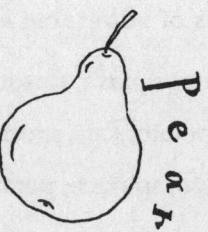

Put the oat flakes and raisins in a cereal bowl and just cover with water (don't drown them) and leave to soak overnight in the fridge. This makes the oats more digestible. In the morning mash or purée the oats and raisins and mix with the apple and pear purée.

> **Handy hint**
> To make this more of a meal, add some ground nuts or seeds. It makes a great pudding as well as a breakfast.

Vegetable Bases

To ensure that you are giving your baby an immune-boosting diet, it is a good idea to have a stock of vegetable bases. These are designed so that you can just add some protein at the last minute. The list opposite should only be regarded as examples, because by this stage you will undoubtedly have got the hang of purées and probably be overflowing with them! To make a good immune-boosting vegetable base choose a red, yellow or orange vegetable and a green one. Colourful fruits and vegetables are rich in antioxidants, which are excellent for building a strong immune system. Steam them, then purée and freeze in individual portions or ice cubes depending on your baby's appetite.

Examples of vegetable bases

- butternut squash, carrot, parsley and broccoli

- sweet potato, kale, green bean and sweetcorn

- pumpkin, spinach, potato and courgette

- beetroot, potato, parsley and broccoli
- red pepper, sweetcorn, pea and potato
- tomato, potato, watercress and carrot

Suitable protein add-ins are:

- a slice of cooked organic chicken breast
- a teaspoon of hummus
- a teaspoon of cashew butter
- a teaspoon of almond butter
- a slice of cooked organic lamb
- a cooked egg yolk
- a teaspoon of tinned albacore tuna (in oil, not brine)
- a teaspoon of ground almonds
- a teaspoon of ground sunflower seeds or pumpkin seeds
- a teaspoon of tahini
- Chicken Liver Medley (page 126)

Baked potato ideas

Baked potatoes in their jackets are a deliciously easy meal for all the family. By adding fillings containing antioxidant-rich vegetables and plenty of essential fatty acids you can guarantee another quick immune-boosting meal for your baby. The following combinations are so yummy that all the family will soon become addicted. You can make the hummus (see recipe below), while the nut butters, tahini and sprouted seeds can be bought from a healthfood shop or from a mail order company such as Organics Direct (see Resources). You may need to add a little liquid, such as vegetable stock, water or milk, to thin the mixtures.

Baby Hummus

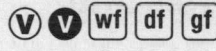

To convert to an adult version and prevent wastage add 1 teaspoon ground cumin seeds and garnish with parsley. This will keep for up to 2 weeks in the fridge. Make sure you use a no sugar, no salt variety of chickpeas.

MAKES 1 SMALL BOWLFUL

1 tin cooked chickpeas
1 clove garlic
1 tablespoon light tahini
6 tablespoons extra-virgin olive oil

Put all the ingredients into a liquidiser or food processor and whizz up until smooth. You may want to drizzle a little more olive oil into the mixture if it is too thick.

Baked Potato, Hummus and Cooked Broccoli

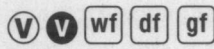

MAKES 1 SERVING

1 small baked potato
1 heaped teaspoon hummus
2 florets broccoli

Bake the potato for 30–45 minutes, depending on size. Steam the broccoli for 5 minutes until soft. Scoop out the potato from the skin and mash with the hummus and broccoli.

Baked Potato, Almond Butter and Sprouted Seeds

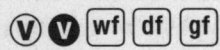

MAKES 1 SERVING

1 small potato
1 dessertspoon mixed sprouted seeds
1 teaspoon almond butter

Bake the potato for 30–45 minutes, depending on size. Meanwhile, finely grind the sprouted seeds in a coffee grinder or liquidiser. Scoop out the potato from its skin and mash with the almond butter and ground sprouted seeds.

Sweet Potato, Tahini and Parsley

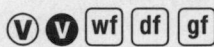

MAKES 1 SERVING

1 small sweet potato
1 teaspoon tahini
1 sprig parsley, washed and finely chopped

Bake the sweet potato for 30–45 minutes, depending on size. Scoop out the sweet potato from its skin and mash with the tahini and parsley.

Baked Potato, Avocado and Pumpkin Seed Paste

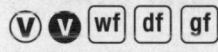

Pumpkin seeds are rich in zinc as well as in essential fatty acids. You can either make your own pumpkin seed paste by grinding the seeds to a pulp, or buy it from healthfood shops. Remember to keep it in the fridge once opened.

MAKES 1 SERVING

1 small potato
1 teaspoon pumpkin seed paste or equivalent of ground
    pumpkin seeds
½ avocado

Bake the potato for 30–45 minutes, depending on size. If using pumpkin seeds, finely grind them in a coffee grinder or liquidiser. Scoop out the potato from its skin and mash with the avocado and pumpkin seed paste. You may need to add a little milk or water to achieve the desired consistency.

Main meals

Barley Stew*

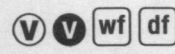

This makes a lovely warming winter dish for all the family. It contains all the foods that help to keep the bugs at bay.

MAKES 2 SERVINGS

1 small onion, peeled and finely chopped
1 clove garlic, peeled and crushed
1 tablespoon extra-virgin olive oil
4 shiitake mushrooms, wiped and thinly sliced
pinch ground ginger
pinch ground cloves
1 organic carrot, washed, peeled and grated
¼ cup pot barley
600 ml (1 pint) vegetable stock *or* 10 cubes frozen vegetable stock (see page 81)
dice-sized cube creamed coconut

In a pan, lightly cook the onion and garlic in the olive oil until transparent. Add the mushrooms and cook for a couple of minutes. Sprinkle in the spices and mix well. Add the rest of the ingredients except the creamed coconut. Simmer gently for 40–50 minutes until the barley is really soft. Once cooked, add the creamed coconut and stir until dissolved. Mash or purée to desired consistency.

Tofu Hotpot*

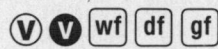

Tofu is the most marvellous source of protein, and since many brands are calcium-enriched it is an excellent dairy alternative for this age group.

MAKES 2–3 SERVINGS

1 tablespoon extra virgin olive oil
1 onion, peeled and sliced
1 tablespoon millet grain
½ pack firm tofu, cubed
1 tablespoon tinned sweetcorn (no sugar, no salt variety)
1 tablespoon frozen peas or fresh peas
1 tablespoon chopped parsley
300 ml (½ pint) vegetable stock *or* 10 cubes frozen vegetable
    stock (see page 81)

Put the olive oil in a pan, add the onion and gently cook until transparent. Add the millet and tofu, and stir well to coat with oil. Add the rest of the ingredients and gently simmer for 15 minutes until the millet is cooked. Mash or purée to the desired consistency.

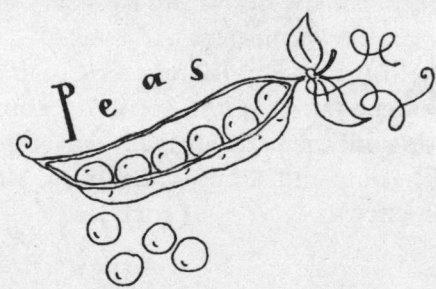

Root Vegetable and Butter Bean Stew*

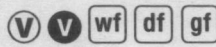

MAKES 3–4 SERVINGS

1 onion, peeled and chopped

1 tablespoon extra-virgin olive oil

450 g (1 lb) organic mixed root vegetables (carrot, potato, sweet potato, turnip, parsnip, swede, celery etc.), washed, peeled and diced

600 ml (1 pint) filtered water

1 tablespoon potato flour

a sprig fresh oregano *or* a sprinkling dried herbs

1 × 425 g (15 oz) tin butter beans (no sugar, no salt variety)

Preheat the oven to 160°C/325°F/gas 3. In a heavy casserole pan gently cook the onion in the olive oil until transparent. Add the vegetables and cover with the water. Mix the potato flour to a smooth paste with a little cold water to prevent lumps, and stir into the casserole. Sprinkle in the herbs and add the beans. Bring to the boil and then bake, covered, for 2 hours. Mash or purée to desired consistency.

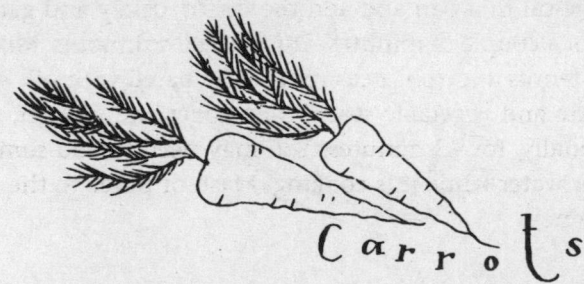

Carrots

Lentil Millet Risotto*

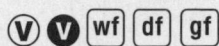

This vegetarian recipe is delicious and contains plenty of immune-boosting nutrients. I love this risotto. It is real comfort food on a winter's day, rich in natural antibacterial agents. Double the quantities in the recipe and it will feed two adults and two teenagers.

MAKES 3–4 SERVINGS

1 tablespoon extra-virgin olive oil
1 organic carrot, washed, peeled and chopped
1 stalk celery, washed and sliced
1 clove garlic, peeled and crushed
4 shiitake mushrooms, washed and sliced
1 tablespoon millet
1 tablespoon green or brown lentils
1 tablespoon dried split peas
1 organic courgette, washed and sliced
600 ml (1 pint) vegetable stock *or* 20 cubes frozen vegetable
    stock (see page 102)

Heat the oil in a pan and add the carrot, celery and garlic and sauté for a couple of minutes. Stir in the mushrooms. Mix in the millet, lentils and split peas until well coated with oil. Add the courgette and vegetable stock, then cover and simmer, stirring occasionally, for 45 minutes. You may need to add some extra stock or water while it is cooking. Mash or purée to the desired consistency.

Chicken Liver Medley*

wf df gf

Liver is packed full of iron and vitamin A, essential for growth and development and for a healthy immune system. As this is a rich recipe and full of fat-soluble vitamins, only serve it once a week. Add to vegetable bases or a scooped out baked potato.

MAKES ABOUT 14 CUBES

1 onion, peeled and chopped
1 tablespoon extra-virgin olive oil
4 organic chicken livers, chopped
4 tablespoons filtered water
4 cubes Dried Apricot Purée (see page 116)
a handful chopped parsley

In a frying pan, sauté the onion in the olive oil until transparent. Add the chicken livers and cook gently until they are cooked through and the juices run clear. Add the water and apricot purée and continue to simmer for 3–4 minutes. Toss in the parsley and cook for another couple of minutes. Purée to the desired consistency.

Salmon and Broccoli Pie*

wf df gf

Salmon is another fish rich in omega-3 essential fatty acids. Make sure you source it well to avoid exposing your baby to unnecessary hormones and antibiotics.

MAKES 3 SERVINGS

1 potato, washed, peeled and cubed
filtered water
small knob unhydrogenated vegetable margarine such as
   Vitaquell
1 small head organic broccoli
1 spring onion, finely sliced
1 tablespoon extra-virgin olive oil
1 skinless, boneless wild salmon fillet, cubed

Place the potato in a pan and cover with water. Cook for 10–15 minutes until soft. Mash with a little margarine and put to one side. Steam the broccoli for 10 minutes until soft. In a pan, gently cook the spring onion in the olive oil for 5 minutes. Add the salmon and keep stirring until it is cooked through. Purée the salmon mixture and broccoli together, adding a little breast milk or formula if needed, and cover with the mashed potato. If you make this in advance, only freeze the salmon mixture as frozen mashed potato doesn't taste very nice.

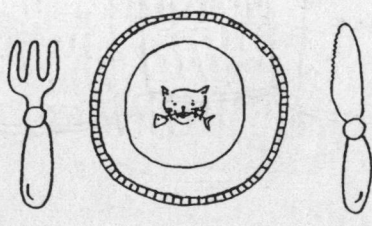

Fresh Tuna and Apple Mash*

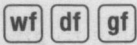

Fresh tuna contains plenty of the omega-3 essential fatty acids which are needed for a healthy immune system.

MAKE 3–4 SERVINGS

1 small onion, peeled and chopped
1 tablespoon extra-virgin olive oil
1 tuna steak, cubed
2 organic eating apples, peeled, cored and chopped
1 organic courgette, cubed
1 large potato, washed, peeled and cubed
a handful parsley, washed
300 ml (½ pint) filtered water *or* 10 cubes frozen vegetable stock
   (see page 102)

Gently sauté the onion in the olive oil in a pan until transparent. Add the tuna and cook for 5–10 minutes until no longer pink. Add the rest of the ingredients, and gently simmer for 15–20 minutes until all the vegetables are cooked through. Purée or mash to the desired consistency, only using as much of the cooking water as you need (if you use it all, it may end up too slushy for your baby's liking).

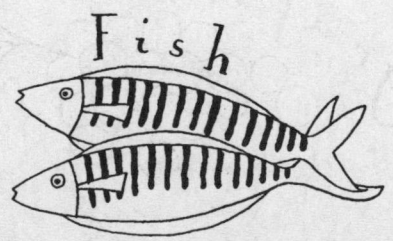

Puddings

At this age, fruit pureés are the most suitable pudding to give your baby. Sugar suppresses the immune system and is therefore best avoided.

Using a banana as a base creates a wonderfully creamy fruit purée. You can then add one of the orange, red, green or blue immune-boosting fruits. Examples include:

- banana and mango
- banana and kiwi fruit
- banana and cantaloupe melon
- banana and apricot
- banana and blueberry
- banana and papaya.

Another healthy pudding is soya yoghurt. You can now buy an organic, live, natural variety which you can mix with some fruit purée from the freezer. Alternatively, you can buy soya yoghurts designed for babies and young children by Provamel called Junior Yofu (see Resources).

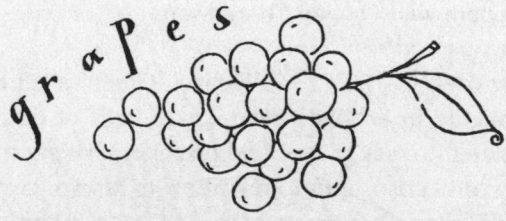

Date Purée

Use in recipes or blend with other fruits. See Oatmeal, Date and Seed Rusks on page 102.

250 g (9 oz) pitted dates (not sugar-rolled)
250 ml (9 fl oz) filtered water

Put the dates and water in a pan. Heat gently for 10 minutes, mashing and stirring all the time, until the dates are soft. Blend to a soft purée. It can be stored in the fridge in an airtight glass jar for up to 2 weeks.

Oatmeal, Date and Seed Rusks

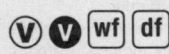

I am really thrilled with this recipe. It has taken me six years to create a wheat-free, dairy-free, sugar-free, rusk-type biscuit that I was happy with!

MAKES 12–14 RUSKS

1 cup oatmeal, medium or fine-cut
1 level tablespoon Date Purée (see above)
1 teaspoon tahini
6 tablespoons warm boiled filtered water

Preheat the oven to 180°C/350°F/gas 4. Combine all the ingredients thoroughly in a bowl. Make small balls of dough in your hands, flatten into rusk shapes and place on a baking tray. Bake for 25 minutes until crisp, and do not allow to brown. Leave for a few minutes to harden, then transfer to a wire rack to finish cooling.

See opposite for weekly menu suggestions.

Weekly Menu Suggestions

	Breakfast	Lunch	Tea
MONDAY	Almond and Rice Porridge (page 114) and pear purée Appropriate milk to drink	Baked Potato, Hummus and Cooked Broccoli (page 120) Fruit pieces	Avocado, banana and tuna Oatmeal, Date and Seed Rusk (page 130) Water to drink
TUESDAY	Millet Porridge (page 97) and apple purée Appropriate milk to drink	Barley Stew (page 122) Soya yoghurt Water to drink	Fresh Tuna and Apple Mash (page 128) Fruit slices Salt-free rice cakes Water to drink
WEDNESDAY	Pear, Apple and Oats (page 116) Appropriate milk to drink	Sweet Potato, Tahini and Parsley (page 121) Mashed banana Water to drink	Salmon and Broccoli Pie (page 127) Blueberry and Apple Purée (page 92) Water to drink
THURSDAY	Banana, Quinoa and Millet Porridge (page 90) Appropriate milk to drink	Tofu Hotpot (page 123) Apple and Molasses Purée (page 94) Water to drink	Chicken and Apricots (page 101) and green vegetable Sweet brown rice pudding Water to drink
FRIDAY	Almond and Rice Porridge (page 114) and peach purée Appropriate milk to drink	Salmon and Broccoli Pie (page 127) Mango and banana purée Water to drink	Fruit slices Water to drink
SATURDAY	Millet Porridge (page 97) and banana purée Appropriate milk to drink	Lentil Millet Risotto (page 125) Soya yoghurt Water to drink	Chicken Liver Medley (page 126) and vegetables Grapes Water to drink
SUNDAY	Cashew, Dried Apricot and Oat Porridge (page 115) Appropriate milk to drink	Vegetable base (see pages 117–118) and 1 teaspoon ground pumpkin seeds Fruit pieces and salt-free corn cracker Water to drink	Banana and kiwi fruit purée Water to drink

Chapter 10

•

IMMUNE POWER FOR TODDLERS – ONE TO FOUR YEARS

Nutrient Focus Chart

Nutrient	Function	Source
Selenium	Antioxidant mineral, which plays a vital role in normal immune function	Nuts and seeds (especially brazil nuts and sesame seeds), wholegrain cereals and seafood
Vitamin E	Antioxidant required for normal antibody function. It works together with other nutrients to build up resistance to infection	Avocados, nuts, seeds, vegetable oils, wheatgerm, oatmeal
Iron	Prevents anaemia and helps the body to resist infection	Dried fruit, spring greens, spinach, parsley, poultry, chicken livers, lamb, red lentils, wholegrain rice

Food for toddlers

Once past the age of one, your toddler will be eating essentially everything that the rest of the family are eating. There are only a very few foods that should not be included at this age, so as to prevent allergies, and that makes meal planning for the whole family really easy. She will be getting more sociable and therefore be exposed to bugs from other children. A strong immune-boosting diet will continue to protect her and help her fight the infections that she will undoubtedly pick up along the way.

It is important that mealtimes are now a family affair. Toddlers and even older children need good role models. This is a time when children learn to feed themselves, to use knives and forks and to have good table manners. If you, or whoever cares for your toddler in the day, eats a sandwich while washing up and doing chores, don't be surprised if you suddenly have a child on your hands who won't sit still at the table and keeps getting up and down. The golden rule for this age group is to sit with the children at mealtimes and eat the same food. Children do what you do and not what you say. If you are sitting down eating and enjoying the same food, you are instilling in your children good healthy eating patterns that will be set up for life. Recent research has also indicated that families who eat together are healthier. If you are preparing a meal for the whole family you are unlikely to serve up fattening, immune-suppressive chicken nuggets and chips!

Drop-offs and parties

Somewhere between the ages of three and four, your toddler will start to be asked out to lunch or to parties unaccompanied. This is an important, fun experience for young children – a great opportunity to help build their confidence and, in relation to food, to make their own choices. Should they come back once in a while having eaten only chips and sweets, just relax. If their immune systems have been built on a strong foundation, a little junk food is unlikely to affect them. It is important, I think, to explain to them why you don't have it at home. Children do need explanations. It is the start of educating them about health, so that they can make wise dietary decisions when they are older.

The only time I would not recommend a visit to a birthday party, either with you or without you, is when they seem a little under the weather or very tired. Sugary food does have a suppressive effect on the immune system, and if they are not feeling great it might be all that is needed to tip them over the edge into illness. Your child will go to many parties in her young life, so she really won't be missing out.

One to four years

Foods to include	Foods to avoid
Fresh fruit including citrus fruits	Strawberries* (introduce age 2)
Dried fruit (unsulphured)	
Grains (oats, barley, rye, wheat*, corn, rice, millet, buckwheat, quinoa, rice cakes)	
Organic poultry, game and meat purées	
Dairy products*	
Fish purées	Shellfish* (introduce age 2)
Soya products (tofu, soya yoghurt, TVP, tempeh, soya cheese, soya milk* (unmodified))	
Nuts and seeds (almonds, cashews, sunflower seeds, sesame seeds, pumpkin seeds, seed pastes such as tahini, peanuts)*	Whole nuts (introduce age 5)
Eggs*	
Honey, malt syrup, fructose, molasses, maple syrup	Sugar (avoid as much as possible)
	Salt (can be used in cooking ingredients, but never add salt to children's food)

The foods marked with an asterisk are the ones most likely to cause an allergic reaction of some kind and therefore their introduction is delayed.

Recipes

These recipes cater for two adults and two children unless stated otherwise. They can, however, very easily be adapted to suit your individual needs by halving or doubling. There are also many recipes in the Five to Twelve Years section which are suitable for pre-schoolchildren. Just check with the chart above for any foods you should not be including at this age.

Breakfast ideas

Muesli Bars

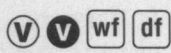

These muesli bars are packed full of immune-boosting minerals and make a really nice change for breakfast. They are also a very good snack food and make excellent emergency breakfast for all the family in the car when you are late on the nursery school run! Fructose, also called fruit sugar, is now widely available from supermarkets. Remember to keep wheatgerm in the fridge to prevent it from going off.

MAKES 12–16 BARS

150 g (5 oz) oatmeal
150 g (5 oz) wholewheat flour
125 g (4 oz) chopped mixed nuts
50 g (2 oz) wheatgerm
pinch cinnamon
2 tablespoons fructose
1 tablespoon molasses
1 tablespoon linseeds
125 g (4 oz) raisins
175 ml (6 fl oz) warm boiled water
75 ml (3 fl oz) walnut oil *or* unrefined sunflower oil

Preheat the oven to 180°C/350°F/gas 4. Mix all the ingredients together in a big bowl with a wooden spoon. Scrape into a lightly oiled baking tin, level the top and cook for 40–45 minutes until golden brown. Cut into squares while still hot and leave to cool. Store in an airtight tin.

Protein-packed Porridge

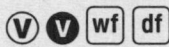 wf df

This delicious combination is packed full of the protein, calcium and essential fatty acids needed for a healthy immune system. I have found it a marvellous way of disguising the taste of flaxseed oil. My children never notice!

SERVES 2 ADULTS, 2 CHILDREN

2 cups porridge oats
filtered water to cover
handful mixed nuts, finely ground
2 tablespoons flaxseed oil
runny honey *or* blackstrap molasses

Place the oats in a saucepan with the water and cook gently for 5 minutes until the porridge has thickened. Turn off the heat, add the nuts and flaxseed oil and stir in well. Serve immediately with a drizzle of raw honey or blackstrap molasses.

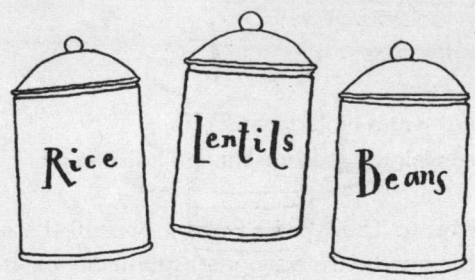

Parsley Eggs

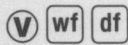

Simple scrambled eggs, transformed with the addition of parsley, make a superfood for the immune system. This recipe is great at breakfast, lunch or teatime. Serve with fresh orange juice for a vitamin C boost and to aid iron absorption.

SERVES 2 ADULTS, 2 CHILDREN

6 organic eggs
a handful chopped parsley
a splash soya milk or cow's milk
a small knob butter *or* Vitaquell Cuisine

Beat up the eggs with the milk and parsley in a jug or bowl. Gently heat the butter or margarine in a non-stick saucepan and, once melted, pour in the egg mixture. Cook over a low heat, stirring with a wooden spoon, for 5–6 minutes until the egg thickens and is cooked. Serve on gluten-free bread, wholemeal bread or Ryvita.

Main meals

Carrot and Orange Soup*

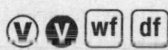

This soup is so quick to make and packed full of carotenoids and other phytonutrients. It will soon become a family favourite. Although it does freeze it tends to go a bit watery – so eat fresh if possible.

SERVES 2 ADULTS, 2 CHILDREN

1 onion, peeled and finely chopped
1 tablespoon extra-virgin olive oil
450 g (1 lb) organic carrots, washed, peeled and chopped
1 teaspoon grated orange zest
600 ml (1 pint) stock made from low-salt Marigold Swiss
    vegetable bouillon powder *or* 12–14 cubes frozen vegetable
    stock (see page 102)
juice 1 orange
organic cheddar cheese *or* soya cheese, grated

In a heavy pan, gently cook the onion in the oil until transparent. Add the carrots and orange zest and continue cooking for 5 minutes to soften the carrot. Pour in the stock and simmer for 20 minutes. Add the orange juice and liquidise. Sprinkle the cheese on top for added protein and serve with wholemeal toast chopped into crouton shapes, baby rice cakes that can float on top or rye crackers.

Toddler Borscht*

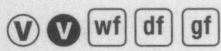

Beetroot has a reputation as a potent immune stimulator. Rich in vitamins and phytonutrients, it makes a healthy and colourful addition to your toddler's diet. Just don't be alarmed if she has pink nappies after eating beetroot. This is a result of her not metabolising the red pigment in beetroot, betacyanin, a harmless substance which just passes straight through the digestive system. In the salad section of supermarkets you can now buy cooked organic beetroot vacuum-packed with water, which makes this recipe much quicker to make than when using raw beetroot.

SERVES 2 ADULTS, 2 CHILDREN

1 onion, peeled and finely chopped

1 tablespoon extra-virgin olive oil

2 ¥ 200 g (7 oz) pack cooked organic beetroot

4 organic carrots, washed, peeled and sliced

3 sticks of celery, washed and diced

900 ml (1½ pints) stock made from low-salt Marigold Swiss vegetable bouillon powder *or* 20 cubes frozen vegetable stock (see page 102)

a sprig fresh thyme *or* a pinch dried thyme

In a heavy pan, sauté the onion in the oil until transparent. Add the beetroot, carrots and celery and continue cooking for 5 minutes. Pour in the stock and add the thyme. Simmer for 30 minutes. If too much liquid evaporates, add a little more stock. Liquidise the soup and serve with wholemeal toast chopped into crouton shapes, baby rice cakes or rye crackers.

Colourful Chips

Ⓥ Ⓥ wf df gf

These are very popular in our house. If you use organic vegetables there is no need to peel them, which also helps to prevent their breaking up (but you should still wash them well). By using colourful root vegetables as well as potatoes you will be giving your child lots of immune-boosting nutrients.

SERVES 2 ADULTS, 2 CHILDREN

2 sweet potatoes
1 potato
1 chunky carrot
1 parsnip
1 tablespoon extra-virgin olive oil for brushing
a sprinkling dried oregano

Preheat the oven to 220°C/425°F/gas 7. Wash the vegetables and cut into chunky chip shapes. Place on a lightly oiled baking tray, brush with olive oil and sprinkle with the oregano. Cook for 45–50 minutes, turning once after 35 minutes.

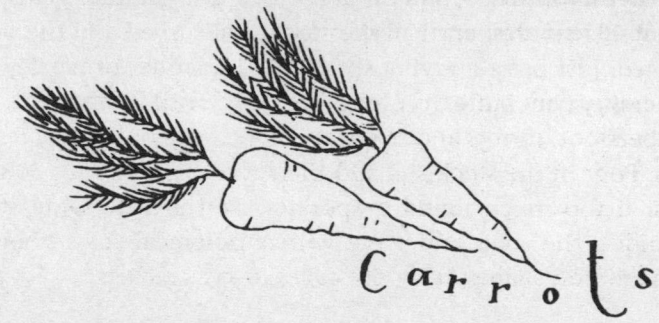

Carrots

Butternut Squash Risotto

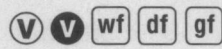

This sweet, dairy-free risotto is an ideal introduction to rice dishes for your toddler. Rich in beta-carotene and antibacterial compounds, it will help to keep your family bug-free through the winter.

SERVES 2 ADULTS, 2 CHILDREN

1 tablespoon extra-virgin olive oil
1 onion, peeled and finely chopped
1 clove garlic, peeled and crushed
1 cup short grain brown rice
1 butternut squash, peeled, deseeded and cubed
900 ml (1½ pints) stock made from low-salt Marigold Swiss
   vegetable bouillon powder *or* 20 cubes frozen vegetable stock
   (see page 102)
a handful chopped coriander or parsley
2 tablespoons cashew nut butter

Place the olive oil in a large frying pan and gently cook the onion and garlic. Add the rice and stir well to coat with the oil. Stir in the butternut squash and stock and simmer gently for about 40 minutes, until all the stock is absorbed and the rice is cooked. Just before serving stir in the coriander or parsley and the cashew nut butter.

Design Your Own Pizza

Believe it or not, pizzas can be healthy. They are also foods that the whole family can get involved in making. Make sure you include lots of the reds, yellows, oranges and purples for an immune-boosting pizza. I have found this recipe is a really good way of encouraging even the most reluctant children to try new things. Semolina flour is available from any Italian delicatessen and from some supermarkets, as is passata.

SERVES 2 ADULTS, 2 CHILDREN

To make the base you will need:
225 g (8 oz) organic superfine wholemeal flour
225 g (8 oz) semolina flour
1 sachet instant dried yeast
175 ml (6 fl oz) warm boiled water
2 tablespoons extra-virgin olive oil
organic passata (sieved tomatoes) *or* tomato purée

Preheat the oven to 230°C/450°F/gas 8. Sieve the flours into a large bowl and discard the excess bran. Make a well in the middle of the flour mixture, pour in the water and oil and tip in the yeast. With a wooden spoon mix it together to form a dough. Once it is roughly mixed, turn out on to a lightly floured surface and knead for 5 minutes. This bit is great fun for the children. Put back in the bowl and leave to one side while you prepare the toppings. Get the children involved and let them choose, for example, one thing from the fridge that they have never tried before and one thing from the larder (see suggestions below).

Divide the dough into two and roll out to form thin pizza bases. Place on a non-stick baking tray. Spread the passata or tomato purée over the base and sprinkle on the rest of the ingredients. Bake for 20–25 minutes until the pizza is crispy and the cheese bubbling.

Topping suggestions

- Thin rings of red onion
- Tinned sweetcorn
- Tinned tuna chunks
- Cooked chicken
- Circles of red and yellow pepper
- Grated carrot
- Grated raw beetroot
- Courgette slices
- Chopped parsley
- Pumpkin and sunflower seeds
- Sprouted nuts and seeds
- Grated cheddar or soya cheese or crumbled goat's cheese or grated mozzarella
- Sliced mushrooms
- Cooked vegetables such as French beans or broccoli florets or peas
- Chopped cooked wild salmon fillet or tinned wild red salmon

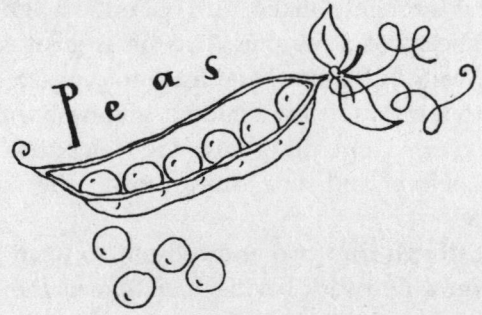

Turkey Burgers

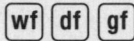

Turkey is a lean white meat which contains over one-third more zinc than chicken. It makes healthy burgers that toddlers love.

MAKES 6 BURGERS

225 g (8 oz) or 2 medium potatoes, washed, peeled, cooked and mashed
1 onion, peeled and finely chopped
1 tablespoon extra-virgin olive oil
a pinch ground cloves
225 g (8 oz) organic minced turkey
a handful chopped parsley

In a pan, gently cook the onion in the olive oil until transparent. Add the cloves and stir well. Add the turkey mince and cook for about 10 minutes, stirring continuously until the turkey is cooked through. Take off the heat, add the mashed potato and parsley and put aside until cooled enough to handle. Then form into small burger shapes and place in the fridge to set for 30 minutes. Brush with olive oil and grill for 5 minutes each side. If you like, you can roll them in sesame seeds before grilling.

Red Lentil and Spinach Lasagne

This vegetarian lasagne has plenty of hidden goodies to boost your child's immune system. By adding the spinach purée, you are boosting the overall iron content of this dish.

SERVES 2 ADULTS, 2 CHILDREN

1 onion, peeled and chopped
1 clove garlic, peeled and crushed
1 tablespoon extra-virgin olive oil
100 g (4 oz) red lentils
600 ml (1 pint) stock made from low-salt Marigold Swiss vegetable bouillon powder *or* 12–14 cubes frozen vegetable stock (see page 102)
1 × 200 g (7 oz) tin sweetcorn (no sugar, no salt variety)
½ × 425 g (15 oz) tin organic no-sugar baked beans
2 cubes spinach purée
8 precooked lasagne sheets
100 g (4 oz) cheddar cheese *or* dairy-free equivalent, grated
handful chopped parsley

Preheat the oven to 180°C/350°F/gas 4. Place the oil in a large pan, add the onions and garlic and sauté until transparent. Stir in the red lentils and coat well with oil. Cover with the stock and simmer for 15 minutes. Add the sweetcorn, baked beans and spinach and simmer for 5 minutes. Put a fifth of the mixture in an oiled ovenproof dish, place some lasagne sheets on top and sprinkle with cheese. Repeat until all the ingredients are used up, finishing with a layer of cheese. Cover with foil and bake for 30 minutes. Sprinkle with parsley and serve with a crunchy salad.

Chicken in a Pot

df

This delicious recipe is so easy to prepare and can be left to cook while you are out and about. The addition of thyme makes it a comforting dish when there are coughs and colds around.

SERVES 2 ADULTS, 2 CHILDREN

1 onion, peeled
1 organic chicken
3 organic carrots, peeled and chopped
10 shallots, peeled
1 litre (2 pints) organic apple juice
a few sprigs thyme

Preheat the oven to 180°C/350°F/gas 4. Stuff the peeled onion in the middle of the chicken then place the chicken in a heavy casserole dish. Surround the chicken with apple juice (enough to go halfway up the chicken). Add the carrots, shallots and thyme, and bake for 1 1/2 hours. Once cooked, remove the excess fat. You can then thicken up the gravy by removing the chicken and vegetables on to a serving dish and stirring in a heaped tablespoon of potato flour or plain flour, mixed with a little cold water, to the gravy. Bring to the boil, stirring, and simmer for a few minutes to reduce. Pour over the chicken. Serve with mashed or baked potatoes and broccoli or spring greens.

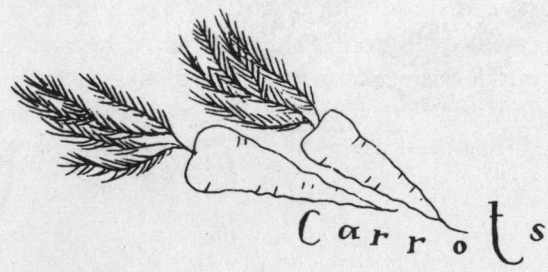

Carrots

Potato Person

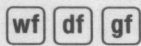

This recipe is a fun way of serving up baked potatoes for a lunchtime or teatime dish. Your toddler will enjoy making these with you.

MAKES 1 POTATO PERSON

1 baked potato per person, washed and scrubbed
1 tin albacore tuna fish or tuna fish in water or oil (not brine)
a handful raisins
1 carrot, peeled and cut into sticks
a handful alfalfa sprouts

Preheat the oven to 180°C/350°F/gas 4 and bake the potatoes for 45 minutes to 1 hour or until cooked. Slice the top off each potato and put to one side. Spoon out the potato from the larger portion and mash it with the tuna. Put the potato mixture back in the skin, allowing it to pile up over the edge. Use 2 raisins for eyes and a carrot stick for a nose. Put the alfalfa sprouts on top as hair and pop the potato hat on the top. A meal in one.

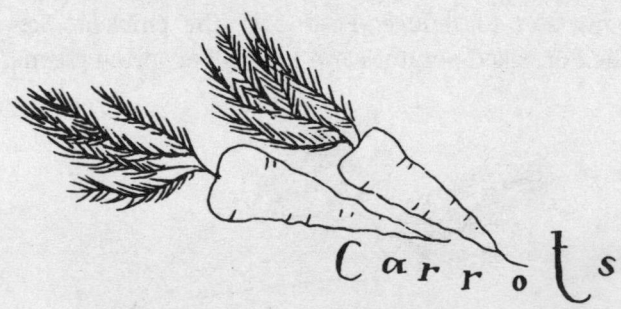

Carrots

Root Vegetable Rosti

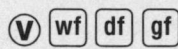

This is a really quick and popular tea. By adding some colourful root vegetables and parsley, you are giving your children plenty of immune-boosting vitamins and minerals. If you have a food processor with a grating attachment, this is really quick – I also find that hand grating doesn't get the vegetables quite thin enough.

SERVES 2 ADULTS, 2 CHILDREN

1 large organic carrot, peeled and grated
1 large organic potato, peeled and grated
1 large organic parsnip, peeled and grated
a handful chopped parsley
1 organic egg, beaten
extra-virgin olive oil for frying

Wrap the grated vegetables in kitchen towel to absorb as much moisture as possible. Mix the vegetables, parsley and egg together in a bowl. Heat the oil in a frying pan or wok. When really hot, drop a tablespoon of the mixture into the pan and flatten slightly. Cook the rosti in batches like this, for 5–8 minutes each side, until they are golden brown. Serve with salad.

Family Fish Pie*

Fish pie is always a family favourite. Here is a variation on the normal theme, achieved by adding some oily fish (salmon and mackerel) to boost the essential fatty acid content. The recipe can be made with milk or dairy-free. Don't add the prawns until your child is over 2 years old.

SERVES 2 ADULTS, 2 CHILDREN

1 large skinless, boneless cod fillet
1 skinless, boneless wild salmon fillet
soya milk or semi-skimmed milk to cover the fish
1 fresh mackerel (without its head or tail) *or* 1 tin mackerel
   fillets in oil
2 organic hard-boiled eggs, chopped
a handful frozen cooked prawns, defrosted
a handful chopped parsley
450 g (1 lb) potatoes, boiled and mashed

Sauce
the milk in which the fish was cooked
1 tablespoon butter *or* unhydrogenated cooking margarine such
   as Vitaquell
2 tablespoons plain flour or gluten-free flour

Preheat the oven to 190°C/375°F/gas 5. Poach the cod and the salmon in the milk for 20–30 minutes. If using fresh mackerel, bake with a drizzle of olive oil and a squeeze of lemon in a separate, covered dish for 20–30 minutes depending on size (tinned mackerel will need no cooking at this stage). Keeping the milk in which you cooked the white fish, flake all the fish carefully and place in a fresh ovenproof dish. Make sure you remove all the skin and bones. Mackerel contains many very small bones, so be particularly vigilant here.

Now make the sauce. Put the milk, butter and flour into a small pan and, using a whisk, beat together vigorously over medium heat until a nice smooth sauce has formed. Chop the hard-boiled eggs and add to the fish dish. Add the prawns. Pour the white sauce on top, add the parsley and mix all the ingredients together. Cover with the mashed potato and bake for 30 minutes until golden brown on top.

Venison Shepherd's Pie*

Being game, venison is lower in fat than other red meat such as beef or lamb. It is also rich in iron, essential for a healthy immune system.

SERVES 2 ADULTS, 2 CHILDREN

1 onion, peeled and chopped
1 clove garlic, peeled and crushed
1 tablespoon extra-virgin olive oil
450 g (1 lb) venison mince
a handful mushrooms, finely chopped
1 organic carrot, peeled and diced
150 ml (¼ pint) Kallo vegetable gravy browning
2 tablespoons tomato purée
450 g (1 lb) potatoes, washed, peeled, cooked and mashed

Gently sauté the onions and garlic in the olive oil in a pan until translucent. Add the mince and brown well. Add the mushrooms and carrots, then stir in the gravy browning and tomato purée. Mix well and simmer for 1 hour, stirring occasionally. Once cooked, scoop off any excess fat. Pour the meat mixture into an ovenproof dish and cover with the mashed potato. Bake in a hot oven for 30 minutes before serving with the family's favourite green vegetable.

Puddings

For toddlers, puddings should be mainly fruit-based. Here are some ideas.

Berry Booster Yoghurt Lollies*

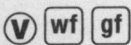

This is a wonderful recipe for making delicious home-made ice cream free from artificial colours and flavours and full of immune-boosting nutrients. For a dairy-free version you could use natural soya yoghurt and add some honey to sweeten it slightly. Yeo Valley do a lovely yoghurt that works a treat in this simple recipe.

MAKES 4–6 LOLLIES

1 pot organic strawberry yoghurt
1 packet frozen berries or fresh in season

Defrost the frozen fruit to room temperature. Whizz up in a food processor and then sieve to remove seeds. Combine the yoghurt with the sieved fruit and pour the mixture into lolly moulds. Freeze until set.

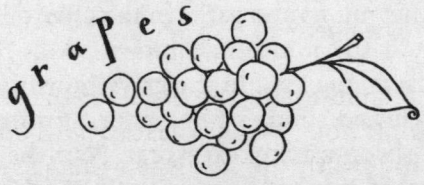

Frozen Banana Ice Cream

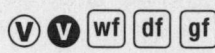

This tastes like the real thing! As it uses just fruit and no sugar it is also incredibly good for your children.

MAKES 1 SERVING

2 bananas per child

Slice the bananas in half lengthwise and place on a baking tray. Put in the freezer for 6 hours until frozen. Bananas never quite freeze, which is why they work so well. Once hard, put through a juicer or liquidiser and eat straightaway.

Yoghurt Mountain

This is a great way of serving natural yoghurt, which is free from sugar and artificial preservatives, colours and flavours. It also contains beneficial bacteria which can offer immune support. Use raw honey if you can find it, as it has antibacterial properties.

MAKES 1 SERVING

150 g (5 oz) pot natural live set yoghurt
1 tablespoon runny honey
1 tablespoon wheatgerm

Carefully run a knife round the inside of the yoghurt pot to release the yoghurt from the sides. Place a bowl upside down on top of the pot and swiftly turn the whole thing over. Holding on to the bowl, shake down gently and then lift off the pot to reveal a mound of yoghurt. Sprinkle the wheatgerm around the bottom of the yoghurt and drizzle the honey over the top.

Bio Yog Pots

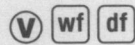

In supermarkets you can now buy really unhealthy double yoghurt pots which have yoghurt one side and fruit in syrup, sweets or sugar-laden cereals the other side. The only relatively healthy one has muesli on one side and natural yoghurt on the other. I buy these and then use the pots to make truly healthy puddings! Put natural live yoghurt in one side (drizzled with honey if you are still converting your child to natural yoghurt) and something nutritious in the other, for instance:

- fresh fruit salad
- raisins
- dried fruit pieces
- sugar-free muesli
- organic cornflakes
- home-made popcorn
- frozen banana pieces

MAKES 1 SERVING

Mango Smoothie

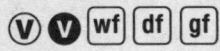

You can combine any fruit with bananas to create smooth fruit puddings that are a lovely alternative to yoghurt. Mangoes are rich in vitamin C and beta-carotene, essentials for a healthy immune system.

MAKES 2 SERVINGS

2 frozen bananas, 1 mango

Slice the mango either side of the (very large) stone and peel the flesh away. In a liquidiser or food processor blend the bananas and mango until you have a beautiful velvety texture. Serve in a bowl immediately.

Mini Raisin Scotch Pancakes with Banana Butter

These are very quick to make and are sugar-free – the raisins and banana are the only sweeteners. Delicious for breakfast or as a pudding.

MAKES 24–36 MINI PANCAKES DEPENDING ON SIZE

1¼ cups superfine wholemeal flour or spelt flour
½ teaspoon bicarbonate of soda
1 teaspoon cream of tartar
1 organic egg, beaten
1¼ cups soya milk or semi-skimmed milk
1 cup sun-dried raisins
2–3 ripe bananas

Sieve the flour with the bicarbonate of soda and the cream of tartar and discard the bits that won't go through (even if it seems quite a lot). Mix in the egg and add the milk slowly to create a batter. (This can be made in advance if you prefer. Make it last thing at night, cover and put in the fridge, and it will be ready to make pancakes for breakfast.) Tip in the raisins and stir well. Drop dessertspoons of the mixture into a very hot, dry, non-stick frying pan. When bubbles appear on top of the pancakes, flip them over to cook on the other side. This can take as little as a minute, depending how hot the pan is. Once cooked, place on a warmed serving plate and do further batches until all the batter is used. Mash the banana in a bowl and serve with the pancakes – which your children can spread on their pancakes themselves.

Mimi's Blackberry Pies

This idea came from a storybook that the boys loved all about Mimi the mouse and her blackberry pies. We would go off to pick blackberries and then come back and make them into pies – that is, when we didn't eat them all on the way home! You can use any berries for this recipe, or use a fruit-based jam if out of season. They are equally delicious.

MAKES 8 PIES

2 cups spelt flour
½ cup ground almonds
2 tablespoons fructose
175 g (6 oz) unhydrogenated margarine
2 organic eggs
24 ripe blackberries or other berries in season
a pot of summer fruit compote (available at supermarkets)

Preheat the over to 190°C/375°C/gas 5. Sieve the flour. Mix the flour, almonds and fructose together in a bowl and rub in the margarine. Beat one egg and mix it in to form a soft dough. Roll out the pastry thinly on a well floured surface, cut into 10 circles and 10 lid circles. Put the bases into a well-greased tartlet tray and fill each with a teaspoon of blackberries and a teaspoon of fruit compote. Beat the second egg. Brush the edges of the tartlet bases with beaten egg, put the pastry lids on and press the edges together. Glaze the top of the pies by brushing with more beaten egg and bake for 20–25 minutes.

Walnut Cookies

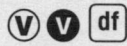

Walnuts are a very good source of omega-3 essential fatty acids. This is an excellent and delicious way of including them in your child's diet.

MAKES ABOUT 15 BISCUITS

220 g (8 oz) spelt flour or superfine wholemeal flour
1 teaspoon baking powder
100 g (4 oz) ground walnuts
100 ml (4 fl oz) raw honey, warmed
100 ml (4 fl oz) walnut oil *or* sunflower oil

Preheat the oven to 200°C/400°F/gas 6. Mix all the dry ingredients together. Add the wet ingredients and mix to form a dough. Form the mixture into small balls, place on a baking tray giving each one space to spread, and flatten with a fork. Bake for 5 minutes. Cool the biscuits on a wire rack.

Nut and Currant Biscuits

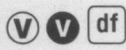

Toddlers will so enjoy helping you make these sugar-free biscuits.

MAKES ABOUT 11 BISCUITS

100 g (4 oz) spelt flour or superfine wholemeal flour
1 tablespoon ground almonds
4 tablespoons currants
½ teaspoon baking powder
½ teaspoon ground cinnamon
50 g (2 oz) unhydrogenated vegetable margarine

Preheat the oven to 200°C/400°F/gas 6. Mix the dry ingredients together. Add the margarine and a little water if necessary, to make a dough. Roll small balls of the dough in your hands, place on a baking tray giving each one space to spread, and flatten with a fork. Bake for 10 minutes. Cool the biscuits on a wire rack.

Nutty Crumble

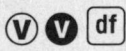

This delicious variation on a crumble is an instant hit with all children, and by adding the nuts you are boosting the nutrient content of the recipe. Doves Farm flour is available from many supermarkets. It is much healthier to grind your own nuts and seeds in a food processor or coffee grinder, rather than buying ready-ground.

MAKES ABOUT 11 BISCUITS

½ cup ground mixed nuts or ground almonds
⅓ cup unhydrogenated margarine or butter
2 tablespoons light muscovado sugar
½ cup stoneground wholemeal flour *or* spelt flour *or* Doves
    Farm gluten-free flour
sprinkle of sesame seeds
7 ripe peaches or nectarines, peeled, stoned and chopped
a handful raspberries or other in-season fruit
1 tablespoon raw runny honey

Preheat the oven to 180°C/350°F/gas 4. Pop all the crumble
ingredients in the food processor and process gently until the
texture resembles breadcrumbs. Do not over-process or you will
be left with a dough. Place the peaches with the raspberries and
honey in an oiled ovenproof dish. Cover with the crumble and
bake for 25–30 minutes.

Handy hint

Other wonderful crumble ideas are blackberry and apple; apple,
raisin and cinnamon; mango and banana; and rhubarb and banana.

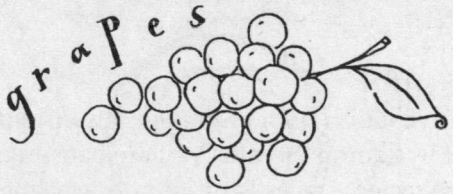

Toddler tea party ideas

On a really large flat serving plate, arrange the following:

- Tiny organic wholemeal sandwiches:
  - Organic cucumber and Marmite
  - Organic almond nut butter
  - Mashed organic egg with a little mayonnaise and chopped parsley
  - Tuna fish and sweetcorn with a little mayonnaise and chopped parsley
  - Organic ham and salad
  - Grated organic cheddar cheese and cherry tomatoes thinly sliced

- Plain popcorn mountain in the middle

- Crudités of cucumber, carrot, peppers and celery around the edge

- Packets of raisins dotted around

- Banana pieces on sticks

- Cheddar cheese cubes and apple cubes on sticks

See opposite for weekly menu suggestions

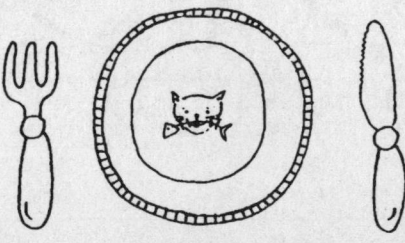

Weekly Menu Suggestions

	Breakfast	Lunch	Tea
MONDAY	Muesli Bars (page 136) Fruit slices Appropriate milk to drink	Butternut Squash Risotto (page 141) Fruit salad Water to drink	Venison Shepherd's pie (page 151) Banana pieces and Walnut Cookies (page 147) Water to drink
TUESDAY	Protein-packed Porridge (page 137) Appropriate milk to drink	Baked Potato, Hummus and salad (page 120) Soya yoghurt Water to drink	Salmon Stir-fry (page 175) Fruit slices Water to drink
WEDNESDAY	Familia Baby Muesli Appropriate milk to drink	Turkey Burgers (page 145) and green beans Berry booster Yoghurt Lolly (page 152) Water to drink	Colourful Chips (page 141) and dips Nutty Crumble (page 158) and custard Water to drink
THURSDAY	Live muesli Appropriate milk to drink	Chicken in a Pot (page 147) with mashed potato and courgette Apple and Molasses purée (page 94) Water to drink	Organic sugar-free baked beans on toast Sweet brown rice pudding Water to drink
FRIDAY	Rice porridge and peach Appropriate milk to drink	Family Fish Pie (page 150) Mango pieces Water to drink	Turkey Burgers (page 145) and broccoli Frozen Banana Ice Cream (page 153) Mini Raisin Scotch Pancakes (page 155) Water to drink
SATURDAY	Millet Porridge (page 97) and banana Appropriate milk to drink	Red Lentil and Spinach Lasagne (page 146) and salad Soya yoghurt Water to drink	Parsley Eggs (page 138) on toast Fruit slices Water to drink
SUNDAY	Parsley Eggs (page 138) and toast Appropriate milk to drink	Venison Shepherd's Pie (page 151) and green beans Fruit pieces Water to drink	Toddler Tea Party (page 160) Water to drink

Chapter 11

•

IMMUNE POWER FOR SCHOOLCHILDREN – FIVE TO TWELVE YEARS

Nutrient Focus Chart

Nutrient	Function	Source
Vitamin A	Powerful antiviral vitamin that strengthens mucous membranes as a first line of defence. Also required for normal thymus activity	Beta-carotene sources: butternut squash, pumpkin, cantaloupe melon, carrots, sweet potatoes, apricots, green leafy vegetables
Vitamin C	Powerful antioxidant which is both antibacterial and antiviral	Citrus fruit, kiwi fruit, peppers, potatoes, blackcurrants, broccoli, Brussels sprouts, papaya, mangoes
B vitamins	The stress vitamins – essential for the development of the thymus gland in infants and for antibody production and phagocytic activity	Liver, yeast, blackstrap molasses, wheatgerm, wholegrains, broccoli, kale, Brussels sprouts, cauliflower, watercress, pulses, nuts and seeds

Once your child reaches full-time school age, somewhere between the ages of four and a half and five, her immune base should be rock-solid. She will pick up colds and bugs at school, but they will not be debilitating and will seldom require her to have time off at home.

From this age, your child will be becoming more independent and making many more choices for herself. She will decide who her friends will be, what foods she likes and does not like, what toys she likes to play with and collect, whether she likes using felt tips or crayons, and whether she likes to wear nighties or pyjamas at bedtime!

During the day she will now be having one meal and one snack at school (more if she attends an after-school club). You may be preparing snacks and packed lunches for her to take, or she may be eating school meals. Feeding your child at this age becomes a bit of a juggling act. Meals, as ever, need to be quick to prepare and tempting to this age group. All school-age children love pasta and I have therefore included lots of healthy pasta recipes which are good for building strong immune systems. Most school food is renowned for being poor in both taste and nutritional content, so it is important to make breakfast and supper nutrient-rich meals.

Whether your child is five or twelve the school day is a long one, so the food they eat must be able to sustain their energy right through the day. For this reason I highly recommend that breakfast contains some kind of protein, for instance:

- ground nuts and seeds added to porridge
- a boiled egg and toast
- scrambled eggs
- toast and peanut butter
- banana and yoghurt

The balance between carbohydrate and protein is one of the lynchpins for sustainable energy. Wholegrains such as oats, wholemeal bread, wholegrain pasta, brown rice and rye also help to ensure that your child does not experience energy dips throughout the day. You can always tell if your children have had a poor lunch full of refined carbohydrates and sugar. When you pick them up from school at 3.30 p.m. are they practically falling asleep or irritable, only to be revived by a quick snack in the car? A diet full of sugar and refined foods will not only suppress their immune systems, it will also diminish their productivity at school.

Opposite is a chart which shows the speeds at which different foods are converted into glucose by the body and released into the bloodstream to produce energy. Wholegrains, foods full of fibre and foods that contain protein, carbohydrate and fibre have the lowest glycaemic index. These are the foods to concentrate on in your school-age child's diet. They will help maintain an even blood sugar level which will optimise her immune function, help her concentration and sustain her energy throughout the day. Get used to checking your meal plans for the week in your mind. Are protein, complex carbohydrate and fibre included in each meal? If, for example, your child's favourite packed lunch sandwich is Marmite and cucumber, add a Babybel cheese or a fruit and nut bar or a handful of seeds as a form of protein, and a piece of fruit, or make the sandwich from wholemeal bread for the fibre (see page 151 for ideas for packed lunches).

The glycaemic index (GI) of foods

How fast are different foods converted to glucose in the body? The higher the GI score (between 0 and 100) the greater and faster the effect on blood sugar levels. The best foods for your child are those that score under 50. Mix higher-scoring foods with lower-scoring foods to create balance.

Low GI foods		Medium GI foods		High GI foods	
Soya beans	15	Buckwheat	55	Mars bar	68
Fructose	20	Popcorn	55	White bread	71
Lentils	25	Basmati rice	55	White rice	72
Kidney beans	29	Sweetcorn	55	Puffed wheat	74
Butter beans	31	Muesli	56	Weetabix	75
Skimmed milk	32	Mangoes	56	Sweet biscuits	79

Low GI foods		Medium GI foods		High GI foods	
Chickpeas	33	Potatoes	57	Instant potato	80
Yoghurt	36	Apricots	57	Cornflakes	80
Pears	37	Brown rice	58	Lucozade	95
Haricot beans	38	Papaya	58	Maltose	100
Apples	38	Honey	58	Glucose	100
Oranges	40	Beetroot	64		
Baked beans (no sugar)	40	Raisins	64		
Wholemeal pasta	42	Sugar	64		
Rye bread	46	Ryvita	65		
Porridge oats	49	Croissant	67		
Carrots	49				
White spaghetti	50				
Peas	51				
Oatcakes	53				
Kiwi fruit	53				
Bananas	54				
Sweet potatoes	54				

Eating 'five a day'

Encouraging your children to eat five portions of fruit and vegetables a day can be really easy if you follow a few of these tricks.

- **At breakfast always have some fruit on the table**, such as melon slices, apple quarters or sliced banana on top of muesli.

- **Always have fruit in the car.** School journeys are often long and boring. This is the time when my children tuck into fruit. In this way, they are making the choice to eat fruit and you are not having to say at mealtimes, 'When you've had your fruit you can have ....' The bonus is that they are learning to snack on fruit and not on junk.

- **When your children are watching a video or television**, I'm sure you find that they get nibbly. This is the time when

I make mine a bowl of mixed fruit pieces or crudités (see page 188). They will often crunch their way through a packet of no salt rice cakes as well. As long as it is not crisps, biscuits or sweets, then I'm happy! Give them diluted juice, soya or rice milk to drink and not packaged fruit drinks full of colours, sugars and preservatives.

Recipes

All the recipes in this chapter serve two adults and two childen unless stated otherwise.

Getting children off to school

Breakfast time can be enormously stressful for both parents and children, especially in a large family when, if you are anything like us, you are always late and can never find the things that need to go to school that day! So here are some quick recipes that can be given to the whole family.

Quick and easy breakfast ideas
- Muesli and banana
- Boiled egg and wholemeal toast soldiers
- Muesli Bars (page 136)
- Fresh fruit salad, natural yoghurt and cereal
- Porridge (pages 97 and 137).
- Wholemeal toast and nut butter
- Baked beans on toast

Blueberry Pancakes

These make a wonderful quick breakfast. You can even make the batter the night before and leave it in the fridge overnight. Blueberries are a good source of vitamin C and contain anthocyanins (compounds which are particularly effective against some forms of *E. coli* bacteria). If your children don't like blueberries, try the Mini Raisin Scotch Pancakes on page 155.

MAKES ABOUT 16–20

1¼ cups wholemeal plain flour
½ teaspoon bicarbonate of soda
1 teaspoon cream of tartar
1 organic egg
1¼ cups soya milk or semi-skimmed milk
1 tablespoon maple syrup
1 punnet blueberries

Sieve the flour, bicarbonate of soda and cream of tartar and discard the bran. Add the egg and stir in well. Slowly add the milk, stirring, to create a batter. Add the maple syrup and mix well. Wash the blueberries and add them. Get your non-stick frying pan very hot, then drop in a tablespoon of the batter. You do not need any oil or butter for cooking. You can probably do 4–5 at the same time if your frying pan is fairly large. When bubbles appear on one side, it is time to turn the pancakes over. Cook for a couple more minutes. Serve plain or with a little extra maple syrup.

Poached Eggs on Toast with Passata

Another great breakfast dish, rich in iron and the antioxidant lycopene which is found in the tomatoes. It would also be good at teatime. Passata is just sieved tomatoes and can be bought in tins or jars from most supermarkets – buy organic if possible.

SERVES 2 ADULTS, 2 CHILDREN

4 organic eggs
4 tablespoons passata
4 pieces wholemeal toast *or* gluten-free toast (page 249)
a little butter
freshly ground black pepper and herb salt, to taste

Boil a pan of water, then turn the heat down so the water is just gently bubbling. Break the eggs one at a time into the water. Cook for 3–6 minutes, depending on how the family like them. Butter the toast, spread the passata on it and place the egg on top. Serve with some freshly ground black pepper and herb salt (available at healthfood shops).

Pasta

All children love pasta. However, most of it is white and made of wheat. As wheat is one of the most common allergens in children, I suggest that you rotate the pastas that you serve. Most supermarkets now also sell brown pasta, which is the better wheat pasta as it is higher in nutrients and fibre than its white cousin. You can also buy rice pasta, rice noodles, corn pasta, buckwheat pasta and barley pasta, as well as some more weird and wonderful varieties from healthfood shops. Remember that they all cook differently, so follow the instructions on the packet carefully and don't overcook them or they will go mushy and disgusting. My children are now very used to the different types, rice pasta penne being their favourite.

Courgette and Garlic Pasta

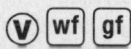

This deliciously simple pasta sauce is easy to prepare, and with all the garlic is a marvellous bug-beater. The amount of pasta you need will depend on your family's appetite.

SERVES 2 ADULTS, 2 CHILDREN

4–6 courgettes, washed and finely sliced
4 cloves garlic, peeled and sliced
2 tablespoons extra-virgin olive oil
225–350 g (8–12 oz) rice spaghetti *or* corn spaghetti *or* fresh
    linguini
a handful chopped fresh herbs
small bowl freshly grated Parmesan cheese *or* cheddar cheese

Put the pasta on to boil while you are preparing this sauce, as it does not take very long and is best eaten straightaway. In a large frying pan, cook the courgettes and garlic with the olive oil. Simmer for 5 minutes until the courgettes are transparent and cooked. Drain the cooked pasta, place in a serving bowl, cover with the courgette mixture, sprinkle the herbs and cheese on top and serve immediately.

Chicken, Basil, Corn and Pea Pasta

wf df gf

I have yet to find a child who does not like this pasta combination. It is colourful, full of immune-boosting nutrients and a really good way of getting flaxseed oil into them – with all the other flavours they just don't notice it! I normally use leftover chicken from a roast. Serve hot in winter, cold in summer.

SERVES 2 ADULTS, 2 CHILDREN

2 organic chicken breasts or leftover chicken from a roast
2 cups frozen peas
a small tin sweetcorn (no sugar, no salt variety)
a handful basil, shredded
2 tablespoons flaxseed oil
rice penne or other suitable pasta

If using raw chicken, grill, griddle or bake until cooked. Cut into small wedges (whether using hot or cold chicken) and put to one side. Put the pasta on to cook. Steam the peas for 5–10 minutes until cooked. Add the sweetcorn to warm through. Mix all the ingredients together and serve immediately with some salad, or refrigerate and serve cold.

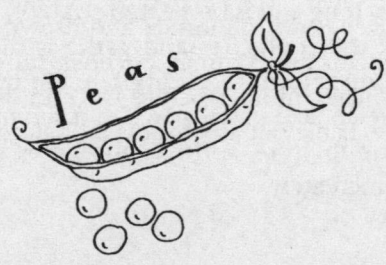

Lamb Bolognese*

wf df gf

Lamb mince is often leaner and therefore preferable to beef mince. Buy organic to ensure you are getting antibiotic and hormone-free meat, which has a much better flavour as well as being healthier (see Resources for mail order suppliers). Adding immune-boosting vegetables such as shiitake mushrooms and spinach makes this recipe a cracker. It is also very good to cook in bulk and freeze.

SERVES 2 ADULTS, 2 CHILDREN

1 large onion, peeled and chopped
1 clove garlic, peeled and crushed
1 tablespoon extra-virgin olive oil
a handful shiitake mushrooms, finely chopped
450 g (1 lb) lean lamb mince
2 organic carrots, peeled and diced
1 × 400 g (14 oz) tin tomatoes (no sugar, no salt variety)
1 heaped tablespoon tomato purée
2 cubes spinach purée (if you have any in the freezer)

In a saucepan gently cook the onion and the garlic in the olive oil until translucent. Add the mushrooms, and cook for a couple of minutes to soften. Add the mince and brown well. Add the rest of the ingredients and simmer, covered, for one hour, stirring occasionally. Five minutes before the end of cooking, add the spinach purée. Ladle out any excess fat before serving.

Roasted Nut and Vegetable Couscous

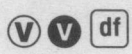

Here is a vegetarian alternative for a couscous dish. This is really good, too, and rich in those all-important essential fatty acids.

SERVES 2 ADULTS, 2 CHILDREN

1 tablespoon extra-virgin olive oil
4 organic courgettes
5 mini aubergines
1 red pepper
1 green pepper
2 red onions, peeled
4 cloves garlic, peeled
1 tin cherry tomatoes or 3–4 fresh cherry tomatoes
a handful basil
2 portions ready-cooked couscous
1 litre (2 pints) stock made from low-salt Marigold Swiss
    vegetable bouillon powder
1 tablespoon poppy seeds
a handful chopped parsley
2 handfuls chopped walnuts *or* cashews *or* sunflower and
    pumpkin seeds, lightly roasted

Preheat the oven to 220°C/425°F/gas 7. Chop the vegetables but leave the garlic cloves and cherry tomatoes whole. Place on a baking tray, scatter with shredded basil and cover lightly with olive oil. Bake for 1 hour until brown around the edges and sticky. Soak the couscous in the hot vegetable stock for 5 minutes, then drain and pile in a large flat serving dish. Add the poppy seeds and parsley for colour. Pile the vegetables on top, and sprinkle the roasted nuts and seeds over the top of everything.

Variation

For meat-eaters, serve the couscous with chicken drumsticks brushed with olive oil and griddled on a high heat for 25–30 minutes, turning regularly until cooked through.

Pasta with Sweetcorn, Carrots and Raisins

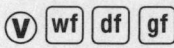

All ages will enjoy this lovely summer pasta dish that is delicious cold – perfect for a picnic or popped in a packed lunch.

SERVES 2 ADULTS, 2 CHILDREN

corn pasta shells
4 organic carrots, peeled and finely grated
2 handfuls raisins
1 small tin sweetcorn (no sugar, no salt variety)
a little chopped parsley
a little salad dressing (see page 217)

Cook the pasta and allow to cool. Mix in all the other ingredients and serve with a green salad.

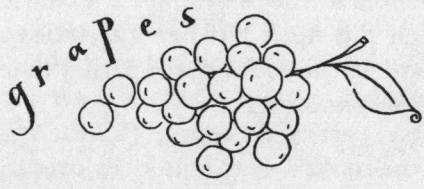

Chicken Risotto

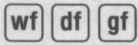

This wonderful risotto is a meal in one, with plenty of immune-boosting vegetables. If you use brown rice you will not have to sit and watch it in the way that you do if you use traditional Arborio rice.

SERVES 2 ADULTS, 2 CHILDREN

2 organic chicken breasts or leftover chicken from a roast
1 onion, peeled and chopped
1 clove garlic, peeled and crushed
2 tablespoons extra-virgin olive oil
1 cup easy-cook brown rice
1 small tin sweetcorn (no sugar, no salt variety)
3 tablespoons frozen or fresh peas
6 mushrooms, washed and chopped
1 courgette, washed and diced
1 small red pepper, deseeded and diced
600 ml (1 pint) stock made from low-salt Marigold Swiss
    vegetable bouillon powder
a handful fresh coriander *or* parsley

If using raw chicken, grill or griddle until cooked, then dice and put to one side. (If using leftover chicken, add at the end with the coriander.) In a large pan gently cook the onion and garlic in the olive oil until transparent. Add the chicken and rice and coat with oil. Toss in the vegetables and add the stock. Cook gently until all the stock has been absorbed and the rice is cooked. Then stir in the coriander or parsley (plus diced left over chicken, if using) and serve.

Salmon Stir-fry

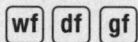

This is a particular favourite in our house. We always use chopsticks for stir-fries, and if you use rice noodles (available in supermarkets) it is easier to eat for the little ones of the family.

SERVES 2 ADULTS, 2 CHILDREN

2 chunky spring onions, sliced
1 clove garlic
1 tablespoon extra-virgin olive oil
2 boneless, skinless wild red salmon fillets, cubed
1 individual portion Sharwood's dried rice noodles
2 handfuls bean sprouts
a packet pak choi, thinly sliced
1 tablespoon honey
1 tablespoon tamari soy sauce

Cook the garlic and spring onions in the oil in a wok (or large frying pan). Add the salmon and stir-fry for 5 minutes or until it turns opaque. Soak the rice noodles in boiling water for 4 minutes. Add the pak choi, along with the other vegetables, the honey and soy sauce, and stir-fry for a couple of minutes. Drain the noodles well, add to the work and stir thoroughly to distribute.

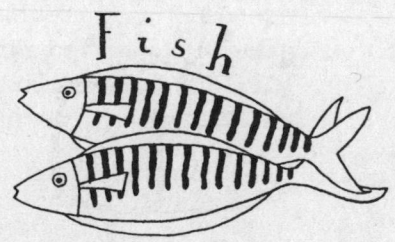

Almond Tofu Stir-fry

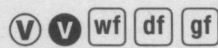

This tofu is fantastic, with a really great flavour. Made by Taipan and available from Waitrose, it is definitely the nicest I have ever found. Even an avid meat eater will enjoy this recipe.

SERVES 2 ADULTS, 2 CHILDREN

1 clove garlic, peeled and crushed
1 onion, peeled and sliced
1 tablespoon extra-virgin olive oil
1 packet smoked almond tofu
1 red pepper, sliced
1 yellow pepper, sliced
1 packet sugar snaps or mangetout
1 organic carrot, peeled and grated
1 tablespoon raw honey
1 tablespoon tamari soy sauce

In a wok, stir-fry the garlic and onion in the oil for a couple of minutes. Cube the tofu, add and toss around in the onion, garlic and oil. Add the rest of the vegetables and stir-fry for 2–3 minutes. Pour in the soy sauce and honey, and continue to stir-fry until the vegetables are well coated in the mixture. Serve with brown rice, millet or quinoa.

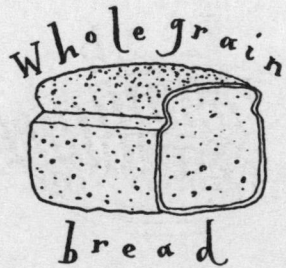

Kedgeree

wf df gf

Another fish dish that is a winner. You can add some vegetables to make it a complete meal, or just serve with a green vegetable such as broccoli or a crunchy green salad. It can be made the night before, or in the morning for a supper dish.

SERVES 2 ADULTS, 2 CHILDREN

1 skinless, boneless undyed smoked haddock fillet
soya milk *or* semi-skimmed milk to cover the fish
1 cup brown rice
2 organic eggs
a handful parsley
a little butter or unhydrogenated margarine

Preheat the oven to 190°C/375°F/gas 5. In an ovenproof dish bake the haddock in the milk for 20–30 minutes until cooked. Meanwhile cook the rice and hard-boil the eggs. Once cooked, drain the fish and discard the milk. Flake the fish. In another ovenproof dish mix the fish, rice, chopped eggs and parsley. Dot with butter or unhydrogenated margarine and bake for 20 minutes until heated through. Serve with a green vegetable or crunchy salad.

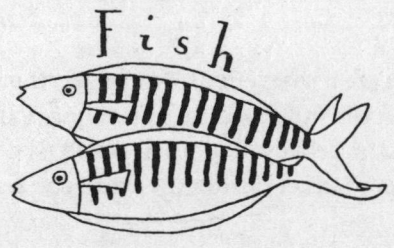

Sesame Fish Fingers

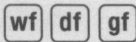

This healthy recipe can be made with any firm fish. The sesame seeds add essential fatty acids and fibre to this wheat-free recipe. If they are unpopular you can substitute breadcrumbs, wheat-free if necessary. Serve with sugar-free, wheat-free tomato ketchup for a good dose of the phytonutrient lycopene.

SERVES 2 ADULTS, 2 CHILDREN

2 chunky skinless, boneless cod fillets
1 tablespoon potato flour or rice flour
1 organic egg, beaten
6 tablespoons sesame seeds
extra-virgin olive oil

Cut the cod into strips. Roll them in flour, then beaten egg, then sesame seeds. Lightly fry in the oil for 5–10 minutes until the fish is cooked through. Serve with Colourful Chips (see page 141) and a green vegetable.

Fish Kebabs

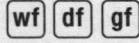

These kebabs are a marvellous way of serving fish to children. If you start with the milder-tasting fishes you can then move on to more elaborate kebabs. Wooden kebab skewers are available from any supermarket during the barbecue season.

SERVES 2 ADULTS, 2 CHILDREN

2 chunky salmon fillets
2 cod or monkfish fillets
12 cherry tomatoes *or* other vegetables e.g. sliced peppers
1 tablespoon tamari soy sauce

Cut all the fish into roughly 2.5 cm (1 inch) cubes. Place on the skewers, with cherry tomatoes at strategic intervals. Brush with soy sauce and grill for 4 minutes each side until cooked through. Serve with a green vegetable and brown rice, millet or quinoa.

Vegetable Kebabs

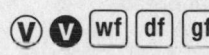

Here is a vegetarian kebab with plenty of brightly coloured vegetables full of phytonutrients for a healthy immune system.

SERVES 2 ADULTS, 2 CHILDREN

225 g (8 oz) block firm organic tofu
8 cherry tomatoes
2 courgettes
4 button mushrooms
½ red pepper, deseeded
½ yellow pepper, deseeded
½ red onion, peeled
1 tablespoon tamari soy sauce
1 tablespoon extra-virgin olive oil

Cut the tofu and vegetables into chunky cubes (but leave the mushrooms and tomatoes whole). Slide a representative mixture of chunks on to each skewer. Brush with soy sauce and olive oil and grill for 3–4 minutes each side, until the vegetables are turning brown at the edges. Serve with brown rice.

Fresh Tuna and Sesame Balls*

df

Fresh tuna is a good source of essential fatty acids which are important for building strong immune systems. Tinned tuna fish, although a very convenient store cupboard food, contains very little, if any.

SERVES 2 ADULTS, 2 CHILDREN

1 large or 2 small fresh tuna steaks
a small bunch spring onions, washed and trimmed
a handful watercress
breadcrumbs made from 4 pieces thin wholemeal bread
2 tablespoons tamari soy sauce
2–3 tablespoons sesame seeds
3–4 tablespoons extra-virgin olive oil

In a food processor, whizz up the tuna steak with the watercress and spring onions to form a paste. Put into a mixing bowl with the breadcrumbs and soy sauce. Place in the fridge to chill for 30 minutes. When chilled, form the mixture into small balls in your hands. Roll the balls in the sesame seeds. Gently fry the balls in the olive oil for about 10 minutes until cooked through. Alternatively you can grill them, but you will need to turn them frequently to avoid burning the sesame seeds.

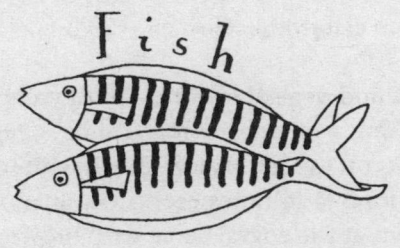

Chickpea and Coconut Curry

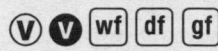

This extremely mild vegetarian curry is a great introduction to the world of immune-boosting spices for the younger members of the family.

SERVES 2 ADULTS, 2 CHILDREN

2 onions, peeled and finely chopped

2 tablespoon extra-virgin olive oil

½ teaspoon turmeric

1 teaspoon ground coriander

4 cloves

2 teaspoons grated fresh ginger

5 cm (2 inch) piece cinnamon stick

3 bay leaves

1 tin chopped tomatoes

1 tablespoon honey

1 tin chickpeas (no sugar, no salt variety)

5 cm (2 inch) cube creamed coconut

In a pan, gently cook the onions in the olive oil. Add the spices and bay leaves and cook for a couple of minutes, stirring well. Add the tomatoes, honey and chickpeas and simmer gently for 5 minutes. Remove the cloves, bay leaves and cinnamon stick. Just before serving add the creamed coconut and stir until dissolved. Serve with brown rice and a range of chutneys and relishes.

Puddings

I have found with this age group that variety is really important. Fruit needs to be interestingly displayed if it is to play a part at mealtimes rather than just be seen as a snack. Some of the suggestions are screamingly obvious, but I have been told by many mothers that it is nice to be given lots of ideas. I have also included a few healthy alternatives to cakes and biscuits for hungry schoolchildren. My boys often have an insatiable appetite at teatime.

Banana and Mango Fruit Salad

This is a really nice combination.

> 2 bananas, 2 mangoes

Slice the banana and chop the mango into cubes.

Melon Balls

Using a measuring teaspoon or melon baller, scoop half a melon out into bowls as melon balls.

Melon Slices and Raisins

Cut a melon in half, discard the seeds and divide into 6 slices. Add packets of sun-dried raisins to the plate.

Apple and Cheese Sticks

You will need a packet of cocktail sticks.

1 organic apple, cored and cut into chunks
organic cheddar cheese *or* soya cheese, cut into cubes

Spear a piece of apple and a piece of cheese on a cocktail stick and arrange several on a plate.

Pineapple and Grape Sticks

You will need a packet of cocktail sticks.

2 slices fresh pineapple, cut into chunks
a handful seedless grapes

Put a grape and a chunk of pineapple on a cocktail stick and arrange several on a plate.

Mixed Fruit Platter

A mixture of dried and fresh fruit works well, and children can just help themselves.

- apple slices
- pear slices
- fresh dates (not sugar-rolled; Medjool are my family's favourite)
- packets of sun-dried raisins
- banana pieces on sticks
- grapes
- strawberries
- blueberries
- kiwi fruit pieces

Baking

Flapjacks

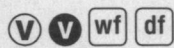

All children love flapjacks. Here is a sugar-free version, using only barley malt syrup and fructose as sweeteners. It works surprisingly well. By adding sesame seeds, you are boosting the protein and essential fatty acid level of this delicious recipe.

MAKES 12 SMALL SQUARES

150 g (5 oz) unhydrogenated margarine or butter
3 tablespoons barley malt syrup *or* corn malt syrup
2 teaspoons fructose powder
175 g (6 oz) oats
50 g (2 oz) sesame seeds

Preheat the oven to 180°C/350°F/gas 4. Melt the margarine in a pan. Add the barley malt syrup and fructose and stir in well. Add the oats and seeds, stir again, and turn the mixture into a lightly greased flat square tin. Bake for 20 minutes. Allow to cool somewhat before cutting into squares, and let them cool completely before removing from the tin.

Sticky Sunflower Balls

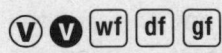

By not using sugar in your cooking you are doing your child's immune system a great favour. This recipe is an interesting and healthy alternative to chocolate krispies. Puffed rice is available at healthfood shops. Children love cooking, and this is one that any age can do.

MAKES 8 BALLS

2 heaped tablespoons barley malt syrup
1 cup plain puffed rice
¼ cup sun-dried raisins
¼ cup sunflower seeds

Melt the barley malt syrup in a heatproof bowl, over a pan of simmering water. In a mixing bowl combine the rice, raisins and sunflower seeds, then pour the syrup over them. Spoon the mixture into paper cases and chill in the fridge to harden.

Honey Cakes

You will need 15–18 paper cases.

MAKES ABOUT 15–18 SMALL CAKES

175 g (6 oz) unhydrogenated margarine or softened butter
125 g (4 oz) raw runny honey, warmed
2 large organic eggs
1 teaspoon vanilla extract
225 g (8 oz) superfine wholemeal self-raising flour *or* spelt flour

Preheat the oven to 180°C/350°F/gas 4. If you have a food processor, mix all the ingredients together. If you are making the cakes by hand, mix the wet ingredients in one bowl and the dry ones in another, then combine and mix well. Spoon the mixture into the paper cases and place in a bun tray. Bake for 15 minutes until golden brown on top and a knife comes out clean when poked into the middle of the cakes. Cool on a wire rack.

Raisin Corn Cake

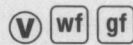 (V) wf gf

This gluten-free cake is delicious served plain or with a little raw honey spread on it.

SERVES 2 ADULTS, 2 CHILDREN

1 organic egg
1 knob butter or unhydrogenated margarine
225 g (8 oz) natural yoghurt
125 g (4 oz) fine cornmeal
1 tablespoon soya flour
1 teaspoon bicarbonate of soda
225 g (8 oz) sun-dried raisins

Preheat the oven to 200°C/400°F/gas 6. Whiz the egg in a food processor until light and frothy. Add the butter and yoghurt and pulse to mix it in. In a mixing bowl sieve both the flours and the bicarbonate of soda. Add the egg mixture to the flour and mix in well. Tip in the raisins, stir in well and scrape the mixture into a well-greased loaf tin. Bake for 30 minutes, until a knife comes out clean when inserted into the middle of the cake. Allow to cool on a wire rack.

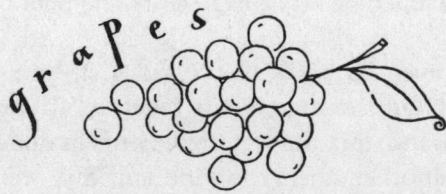
grapes

Banana Yoghurt Cake

This is so quick to make and an instant hit even with the sweet-tooths of the family. The icing sugar is optional and is designed to make it look pretty, not to cover it in a white cloud of sugar!

SERVES 2 ADULTS, 2 CHILDREN

2 small or 1 large ripe bananas
½ cup natural yoghurt
½ cup unhydrogenated margarine
1 large organic egg
225 g (8 oz) spelt flour
⅓ cup fructose
3 teaspoons baking powder
a dusting of icing sugar (optional)

Preheat the oven to 180°C/350°F/gas 4. Combine the banana, yoghurt, margarine, egg and fructose in a food processor until smooth. Add the flour and bicarbonate of soda and pulse until mixed through. Scrape the mixture into a well-greased loaf tin. Bake for 45 minutes to 1 hour until cooked through. Put on a wire rack to cool and sprinkle with icing sugar before serving.

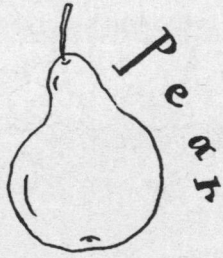

Healthy Snacks

Crudités and Hummus

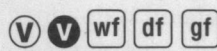

Having a plate of crudités with some plain corn chips and dips ready and waiting when they come back from school is a great way to stop children snacking on crisps and biscuits. It is also a very good way of boosting their antioxidant intake. This hummus is quite delicious and has the added advantage of keeping in the fridge for up to two weeks. If you also have tins of pulses in your larder, this is a brilliant store cupboard recipe which can be made at short notice.

SERVES 2 ADULTS, 2 CHILDREN

1 teaspoon cumin seeds
1 tin cooked chickpeas (no sugar, no salt variety)
2 cloves garlic, peeled
1 tablespoon light tahini
6 tablespoons extra-virgin olive oil

In a pestle and mortar, grind up the cumin seeds to a fine powder. Put all the ingredients in a liquidiser or food processor and whizz up together until smooth. You may want to drizzle a little more olive oil in if it is too thick. Serve with crudités and hunks of fresh bread.

Plate of crudités

- cucumber sticks
- carrot sticks
- celery sticks
- strips of red and yellow peppers
- broccoli florets
- radishes
- pitta bread fingers
- corn chips
- plain tortilla chips

More Healthy Snacks

- home-made tortilla chips and corn chips and dips instead of crisps
- almond butter and crudités
- fruit slices
- Muesli Bar (see page 136)
- Hummus (see page 119) and grissini sticks
- rice cakes with tahini
- corn crackers with almond butter
- nut and raisin mix pack
- fruit kebabs
- Babybel cheese and apple
- fruit smoothies (see page 197)

Healthy alternatives to sweets

In our house, rather than having a sweetie jar, we keep a large jar packed full of fruit and nut bars, dried fruit strips, packets of dried fruit chunks, sesame and honey bars etc. The children love them: they are viewed as treats and seem a really good happy medium between fruit and sweets. Here are some of the brand names I use which are available in healthfood shops and from mail order healthfood suppliers (see Resources). Make sure you look at the ingredients lists and avoid those with added sugar.

- Sun Maid mini packets of raisins
- Whitworth's Frootz, So Very Berry variety (raisins, cherries and cranberries)
- Okanangan fruit snack strips
- Barbara's Nature's Choice cereal bars (wheat-free)
- La Fruit dried fruit chunks
- Shepherd Boy organic fruit and nut bar
- Zaps fruit bar
- Sunita sesame bar with honey
- Hemp 9 bar
- Grizzly bars

See opposite for weekly menu suggestions.

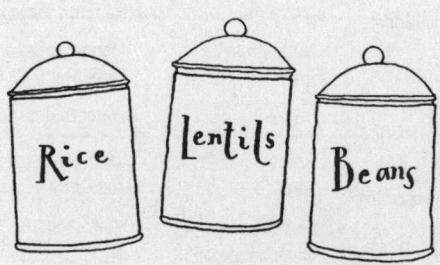

Weekly Menu Suggestions

	Breakfast	Lunch	Tea
MONDAY	Blueberry Pancakes (page 167) Diluted juice or appropriate milk	Packed lunch or school lunch	Chicken, Basil, Corn and Pea Pasta (page 170) Fruit and flapjacks (page 184) Water to drink
TUESDAY	Poached Egg on Toast with Passata (page 168) Diluted juice or appropriate milk	Packed lunch or school lunch	Salmon Stir-fry (page 175) Fruit and yoghurt Water to drink
WEDNESDAY	Organic muesli Diluted juice or appropriate milk	Packed lunch or school lunch	Chicken Risotto (page 174) and salad Fruit and Banana Yoghurt Cake (page 187) Water to drink
THURSDAY	Muesli Bars (page 136) Diluted juice or appropriate milk	Packed lunch or school lunch	Fish Kebabs (page 178) and brown rice Apple and Cheese Sticks (page 183) Water to drink
FRIDAY	Baked beans on rye toast Diluted juice or appropriate milk	Packed lunch or school lunch	Fresh Tuna and Sesame Balls (page 180) Melon slices and Honey Cakes (page 185) Water to drink
SATURDAY	Porridge Diluted juice or appropriate milk	Vegetable omelette and ryvita Nutty Crumble (page 158)	Baked potato and fresh Hummus (page 120) and salad Mango pieces and Sticky Sunflower Balls (page 184) Water to drink
SUNDAY	Croissant (why not!) Diluted juice or appropriate milk	Roast chicken and vegetables Frozen Banana ice cream (page 153)	Sandwich platter with cucumber and carrot sticks and popcorn Fruit smoothie Water to drink

Two weeks of easy, healthy lunch box ideas

- **Monday:** Wholemeal pitta pocket with Hummus (page 188) and cucumber. Carrot sticks. Dried fruit and nut bar. Water bottle.
- **Tuesday:** Chicken, Basil, Corn and Pea Pasta (page 170). Strawberries and a Honey Cake (page 185). Water bottle.
- **Wednesday:** Wholemeal Marmite and cucumber sandwich. Babybel cheese. Tangerine. Sticky Sunflower Balls (page 184). Water bottle.
- **Thursday:** Rice and tuna salad. Melon slices, packet of dried fruit pieces. Water bottle.
- **Friday:** Organic cold cooked chicken and leek sausages. Plain popcorn and vegetable sticks with a dip such as Hummus (page 188), peanut butter dip or vegetable dip. Tub of fruit salad. Muesli bar (page 136). Water bottle.
- **Monday:** Couscous salad (page 172). Flapjack (page 184), banana. Water bottle.
- **Tuesday:** Wholemeal baguette chunk filled with organic ham and salad, mashed egg, grated cheese or leftover chicken. Organic fromage frais. Tub of favourite fruit pieces. Water bottle.
- **Wednesday:** Rice pasta with Pesto (page 202). Mixed salad chunks e.g. celery, cucumber, cherry tomatoes in salad dressing. Fruit and nut bar. Water bottle.
- **Thursday:** Wholemeal bap with almond nut butter and molasses. Vegetable sticks. Yoghurt and a couple of Walnut Cookies (page 157). Water bottle.
- **Friday:** Pitta bread with Fresh Omega-3 pesto (pages 202)and shredded lettuce and cucumber slices. Bag of grapes. Organic sesame seed and honey bar. Water bottle.

Chapter 12

•

IMMUNE POWER FOR TEENAGERS – THIRTEEN TO EIGHTEEN YEARS

Nutrient Focus Chart

Nutrient	Function	Source
Iron	An extremely important mineral required during puberty, especially by girls. It prevents anaemia and helps the body to resist infection	Dried fruit, spring greens, spinach, parsley, poultry, organic liver, red meat, red lentils, wholegrain rice
Magnesium	Magnesium is vital for antibody production as well as for correct functioning of the thymus gland. Low magnesium levels are common in teenagers and may worsen PMS as well as increase allergic reactions	Nuts, seeds, green leafy vegetables, root vegetables, egg yolks, wholegrains, dried fruit
Vitamin E	Antioxidant required for normal antibody activity. It works with vitamin C and other antioxidants to increase resistance to infection and protect from pollution. It is also required to keep skin healthy, a potential problem for teenagers	Avocados, nuts, seeds, vegetable oils, wheatgerm, oatmeal

continues ▶

Nutrient	Function	Source
Zinc	Antiviral antioxidant needed for the growth and development of white blood cells, part of the immune army. It is also required for the maturation of sex hormones, so puberty is an important time to keep well stocked	Poultry, game, lean red meat, nuts, seeds, shrimps, prawns, shellfish, sardines, mackerel, liver, wheatgerm, wholegrains

The teenage years

Between thirteen and eighteen your teenager will go through many changes. The pressure at school will escalate as important exams approach. Their bodies will be changing at a rapid rate as they go through puberty. This is a time when their immune systems are put under extra pressure. Stress can directly suppress the immune system, and it is therefore an important time to give teenagers a nutrient-rich diet which will help them through these turbulent years, boost their immune systems and support their hormonal systems. For this reason the nutrients that I have chosen to feature in the nutrient focus chart will do all these things and are usually the ones lacking in a teenager's diet. If young people go short of these nutrients, deficiency symptoms will occur such as:

- tiredness

- lack of energy

- spots

- increased susceptibility to illness

- constipation

- moodiness.

All the recipes in this section are designed to help combat any deficiencies.

Meals will consist of breakfast at home (unless they are away at boarding school, in which case you will have little control over their eating habits apart from in the holidays). Make sure your teenager has breakfast, even if it is in the form of a shake that you have made for all the family. Lunch will either be packed (see ideas on page 192) or a school meal, and supper will be eaten at home. This will ideally be a family meal, and the recipes in this chapter are designed to feed four adults. Most of them can be eaten by any child over the age of one – just check with the inclusion chart at the beginning of Chapter 10. When you have teenagers you must be prepared to feed unexpected guests at short notice. For this reason I have included lots of recipes that are really quick and can be made from store cupboard supplies.

A note about eating disorders

The teenage years are the most common time for eating disorders such as anorexia and bulimia to raise their ugly heads. Quite apart from the emotional and psychological side of these illnesses, research suggests that a lack of zinc may be an important contributing factor. Zinc is required for taste and smell and a lack of it can destroy the appetite, therefore removing the desire to eat. An obsession with weight and appearance ('Does my bum look big in this?' syndrome) can result in teenagers cutting back on foods that are rich in important minerals such as zinc. Teenagers also often drink coffee and tea and diet drinks, which further strip their bodies of zinc. Making sure that their diets contain zinc-rich foods is an important focus for these years, and regularly checking their mineral status through hair mineral analysis or sweat tests available through nutritionists or nutritionally oriented doctors (see Resources) will help to show whether your teenager is low in zinc and needs a supplement.

Recipes

All recipes serve four adults unless stated otherwise.

Starting the day

Liquid Energy Breakfast

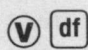

Many teenagers do not like eating breakfast. Here is a delicious liquid breakfast that you can prepare for them before they dash out the door for school. It is packed with all the nutrients they need to support their immune system as well as their hormonal system.

MAKES 600 ML (1 PINT) OR 4 SMALL GLASSES

- 1 cup apple juice
- 1 cup silken tofu or natural yoghurt
- 1 ripe banana
- 1 teaspoon vanilla essence
- 1 teaspoon blackstrap molasses
- 1 teaspoon nutritional yeast
- 1 organic raw egg yolk
- 1 tablespoon wheatgerm
- 1 tablespoon flaxseed oil
- 1 teaspoon lecithin granules

Whizz up in the liquidiser and serve straightaway.

Fruitful

MAKES 1 BOWL

½ banana
½ apple
a few grapes
½ orange
juice of an orange
2 tablespoons natural yoghurt
1 teaspoon raw honey
1 tablespoon sunflower seeds
a sprinkling of wheatgerm

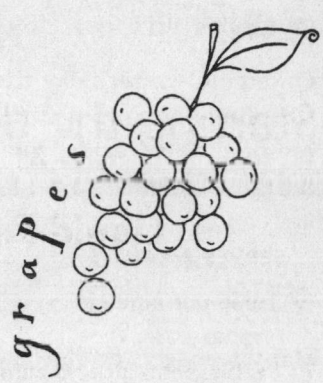

Cut up the fruit and place in a cereal bowl. Pour the juice on top. Spoon the yoghurt over the fruit. Drizzle the honey over the yoghurt and sprinkle with the seeds and the wheatgerm.

Instant Energy Fruit Smoothie

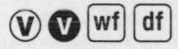

Another quick breakfast drink full of essential fatty acids and zinc, with an extra vitamin C boost to keep the bugs at bay.

**MAKES 600 ML (1 PINT) BUT CAN EASILY BE DRUNK
BY ONE PERSON**

1 cup apple juice
1 ripe banana
1 apple, peeled and cored
a handful of sunflower and pumpkin seeds
a pinch vitamin C powder

Liquidise all the ingredients and drink straightaway.

Pumpkin Seed Porridge

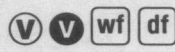

On a cold winter's day there is nothing more delicious than a steaming hot bowl of porridge. Here is one packed with zinc and essential fatty acids, guaranteed to protect your teenager's immune system.

SERVES 4 ADULTS

½ cup porridge oats
filtered water
1 tablespoon ground pumpkin seeds
1 tablespoon flaxseed oil
soya milk or semi-skimmed milk
a drizzle raw honey *or* organic malt syrup

Put the oats in a pan, cover with water, bring to the boil, stirring, and simmer for 5 minutes until thickened and cooked through. Take off the heat and stir in the ground pumpkin seeds. Surround the porridge with a little milk and drizzle with a little honey or malt syrup.

Other great breakfasts for teenagers

- baked beans on toast
- bowl of sugar-free muesli and a banana
- boiled egg and toast with fresh orange juice

Useful stand-bys

Super-immune Chicken Broth

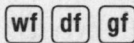

This is really quick to prepare, and fantastic when your teenagers are under par.

SERVES 4 ADULTS

- 1 onion, peeled and chopped
- 2 cloves garlic, peeled and crushed
- 1 tablespoon extra-virgin olive oil
- a small cube fresh ginger, grated
- 8–10 shiitake mushrooms, thinly sliced
- 2 organic raw chicken breasts or equivalent cooked chicken leftover from a roast, cubed
- 1.8 litres (3 pints) stock made from low-salt Marigold Swiss vegetable bouillon powder
- 3 roots pak choi
- 4 individual portions rice noodles
- a handful chopped coriander

Place the onion and garlic in a pan and fry in the olive oil for 2–3 minutes until soft. Add the ginger and mushrooms and cook for a further 2 minutes. If using raw chicken, add to the pan and cook, stirring all the time, until the chicken is cooked and the juices run clear. If using cooked chicken, just add to the pan along with the stock. Shred the pak choi and add, and simmer for 20 minutes. Just before serving, soak the rice noodles in boiling water for 4 minutes, then add along with the chopped coriander. It is fun to eat with Chinese china spoons, which you can find in most cheap wok sets these days.

Quick and Easy Chicken Liver Pâté

Liver is packed full of iron, essential during puberty for growth and development and for a healthy immune system. Chicken livers have a milder taste than lamb's liver, for example, and are therefore usually very popular with all age groups. Only ever use livers from organic chickens, which unlike other chickens reared for food, are not routinely subjected to antibiotics, hormones and growth promoters. The liver of any animal stores drugs and other chemical substances to which it has been exposed, and you could unknowingly be feeding yourself and your children a nasty chemical cocktail. Organic chickens from butchers always come complete with giblets, including the liver (except in supermarkets). If you have an organic source that will supply chicken livers separately, you can increase the quantities in this recipe. But don't add extra garlic cloves because it is not necessary.

SERVES 4 ADULTS

1 large onion, peeled and chopped
2 cloves garlic, peeled and crushed
1 tablespoon extra-virgin olive oil
4 large organic chicken livers, chopped
4 tablespoons sweet sherry
1 tablespoon raisins
a handful chopped parsley
large knob butter or unhydrogenated margarine

Fry the onion and garlic in the olive oil in a frying pan until transparent. Add the chicken livers and cook for a couple of minutes. Add the sherry and raisins and continue cooking until all the sherry has disappeared and the liver has lost its pinkness. Take off the heat, add the chopped parsley and butter and allow to melt, stirring all the time. Whizz up in a food processor until smooth, then pile into a bowl, put a sprig of parsley on top and refrigerate to set. Serve with freshly baked bread and a crunchy salad for a complete meal.

Bruschetta

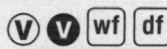

This wheat-free version of the popular Italian recipe works well and provides plenty of immune-boosting nutrients. Village Bakery make delicious rye loaves (see Resources).

SERVES 4 ADULTS

2 cloves garlic, peeled
4 slices thick-cut rye bread, toasted
a handful basil
8 very ripe tomatoes
1 tablespoon flaxseed oil *or* extra-virgin olive oil

Cut the garlic cloves in half and rub them over the toasted rye bread. In a food processor roughly chop the basil and tomatoes with the olive oil. Spoon on to the rye toast and cut in half to form triangles.

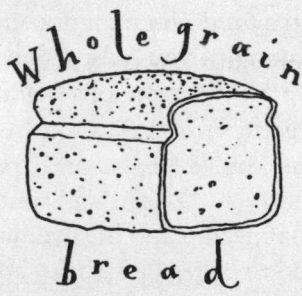

Pasta

Teenagers, I am told, love pasta and some seem to eat nothing else! Here are some slightly more sophisticated pasta recipes for the teenagers in your house.

Fresh Omega-3 Pesto

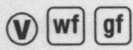

Walnuts are an excellent source of the omega-3 essential fatty acids which are so important for your teenager's immune system. This pesto is very quick and easy to make, so it is very useful when loads of teenagers descend on the house. The rocket gives it a slightly different, sharper flavour, but you can make it with the traditional basil instead if you prefer.

SERVES 4 ADULTS

¼ cup walnuts
¼ cup grated Parmesan cheese
100 g (4 oz) fresh rocket
2 cloves garlic
½ cup extra-virgin olive oil

Grind the walnuts in a food processor or coffee grinder. Add the rest of the ingredients until you have a smooth, slightly grainy paste. You may want to add more olive oil if it is too thick for you.

Smoked Salmon, Spring Onion and Chive Pasta

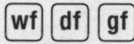

This rather extravagant pasta dish is a wonderful last-minute recipe to prepare for unexpected guests

SERVES 4 ADULTS

1 packet rice pasta spirals or other pasta
a large bunch spring onions, washed and thinly sliced
1 tablespoon extra-virgin olive oil
125 g (8 oz) packet non-farmed smoked salmon, chopped
a handful chives

Put the pasta on to boil. Thinly slice the spring onions and cook in the olive oil for 4–5 minutes. Do not allow them to brown as this will alter their flavour. Chop the salmon, add to the spring onions and stir well for a couple of minutes. When the pasta is cooked, drain and place in a big serving bowl with the salmon and spring onion mixture on top. Finally, snip the chives into little pieces and scatter over the top to make it look pretty.

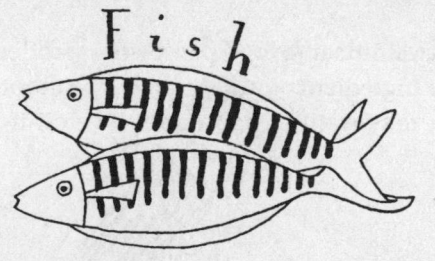

Pasta with Clams

Clams are rich in zinc and selenium, but make sure that you rinse them really well as they are canned in brine and therefore contain quite a lot of salt. Alternatively you can use fresh clams – if your family are happy to cope with shells!

SERVES 4 ADULTS

wholewheat spaghetti *or* other suitable pasta
1 onion, peeled and chopped
1 clove garlic, peeled and crushed
1 tablespoon extra-virgin olive oil
1 tin clams in brine
1 × 400 g tin (14 oz) chopped tomatoes (no sugar, no salt variety)
a handful chopped basil (optional)
Parmesan cheese for sprinkling (optional)

Put the pasta on to boil. Meanwhile, fry the onion and garlic in a pan in the olive oil. Add the clams and tomatoes and simmer for 5–10 minutes. Drain the cooked pasta, pour the sauce on top, and sprinkle with basil and Parmesan if desired.

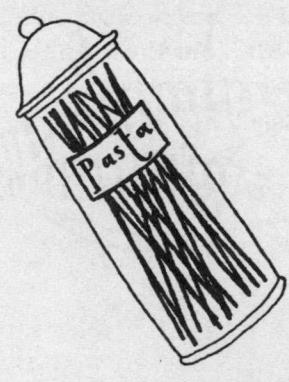

Family Macaroni Cheese

This variation incorporates vegetables and garlic, a true super-food for the immune system.

SERVES 4 ADULTS

175 g (6 oz) wholewheat macaroni
2 spring onions, thinly sliced
1 clove garlic
1 tablespoon extra-virgin olive oil
125 g (4 oz) button mushrooms, thinly sliced
1 tablespoon plain flour
300 ml (½ pint) soya milk *or* semi-skimmed milk
4 ripe tomatoes, skinned and chopped
125 g (4 oz) Gouda *or* cheddar *or* soya cheese, grated
1 heaped teaspoon Dijon mustard

Preheat the oven to 180°C/350°F/gas 4. Put the macaroni on to boil. Meanwhile, gently cook the spring onion and garlic in the olive oil. Add the mushrooms and allow to soften. Add the flour and then gradually add the milk, stirring continuously as it thickens. Add the tomatoes, grated cheese and Dijon mustard and stir in well until the cheese melts. Add the cooked, drained macaroni and stir well. Pour the lot into a casserole dish and bake until crispy on top. Serve with a green vegetable such as broccoli or a green salad.

Healthy fast food

Quick Nut Burgers*

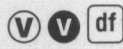

These nut burgers are really quick to make and free from damaged fats.

SERVES 4 ADULTS

6 small slices wholemeal bread
225 g (8 oz) mixed nuts, finely chopped
1 onion, peeled and thinly chopped
1 carrot, peeled and finely grated
1 clove garlic,
1 medium tomato, skinned and chopped
a handful parsley
a few tablespoons sesame seeds
1 tablespoon extra-virgin olive oil, for frying

Put the bread in the food processor and chop to fine breadcrumbs. Tip into a large mixing bowl. Lightly roast the nuts under the grill for a few minutes and then grind finely in the food processor. Add them to the breadcrumbs. Next, chop all the rest of the ingredients (except the sesame seeds) in the food processor, but don't leave the mixture there too long or it will turn to mush. Mix the wet ingredients with the dry ones and form into burger shapes. Roll in the sesame seeds and, with a little olive oil, lightly fry for 5 minutes each side. Keep turning to avoid burning the seeds. Serve with a crunchy salad and sugar-free tomato ketchup, or pop into a pitta bread with some salad and tomato sauce for a packed lunch or picnic.

Minty Lamburgers

These healthy burgers are free from artificial additives, preservatives and colourings and full of immune-boosting nutrients. If you have very hungry teenagers, you may need to double the recipe.

SERVES 4 ADULTS

1 small onion, peeled
½ red pepper, finely chopped
½ green pepper, finely chopped
1 tablespoon passata (sieved tomatoes)
225 g (8 oz) organic lean minced lamb
1 organic egg, beaten
a handful chopped mint
1 large slice wholemeal bread made into breadcrumbs
1 tablespoon extra-virgin olive oil

Roughly chop all the vegetables in a food processor, them put then in a bowl with the meat and passata. Using your hands, mix in the beaten egg, mint and breadcrumbs. Form into small burgers and fry in the olive oil for 5–6 minutes on each side. Serve on wholewheat open muffins or inside mini pittas, accompanied by a crunchy salad and sugar-free tomato ketchup.

Healthy pizzas

Pizzas are very popular amongst teenagers, so here are some ideas for healthy home-made ones. See also page 143 for a great recipe and ideas for toppings. Home-made pizzas can be quick to make, and are infinitely tastier and much healthier. Teach your teenagers to make their own and you are on to a winner!

Potato Pizza

 Ⓥ wf

A quick and easy, wheat-free, pizza base.

SERVES 4 ADULTS

4 large organic potatoes
4 tablespoons extra-virgin olive oil
ripe plum tomatoes
cheddar *or* Mozzarella *or* goat's cheese *or* feta *or* soya cheese
dried oregano
a few olives
any other toppings desired

Grate the potatoes and drain on kitchen towel to remove the excess juices. Heat the oil in a frying pan, put a quarter of the grated potato in the pan and flatten it out into a pizza shape. Cook for a few minutes until the base is brown and crispy, then turn over to cook the other side. When cooked, place on a baking tray. One pizza base will feed one person. Cook the rest of the pizza bases in batches. Start the topping with sliced tomatoes. Sprinkle some dried oregano on top, then crumble your choice of cheese on top. Add some sliced olives (and anything else you fancy) and grill for 5–10 minutes, until the cheese has melted and the tomatoes have cooked.

Corn Bread Pizza Base

With allergies on the increase, this is a smashing, easy recipe for a corn pizza base. Make sure your teenagers are not eating too much wheat and dairy products. Variety will increase the nutrient content of their diet and prevent food intolerances creeping up on them.

SERVES 4 ADULTS

2 organic eggs
450 ml (¾ pint) natural yoghurt
1 knob butter *or* unhydrogenated margarine, melted
250 g (9 oz) fine cornmeal
50 g (2 oz) soya flour
1 teaspoon bicarbonate of soda
200 g (7 oz) tin sweetcorn (no sugar, no salt variety)
1 small onion, finely chopped (optional)

Preheat the oven to 200°C/400°F/gas 6. In a food processor, whizz the eggs until light and frothy. Add the yoghurt and melted butter or margarine. Sift the flours and bicarbonate together into a mixing bowl. Stir in the egg mixture, followed by the sweetcorn and the onion (if using). Pour into four well-greased cake tins or quiche dishes (two dishes if you want deep pizza bases) and bake for 25–30 minutes until cooked through. Cool on a wire rack. You can also bake this as a single cake, but if so it will need 45 minutes to an hour.

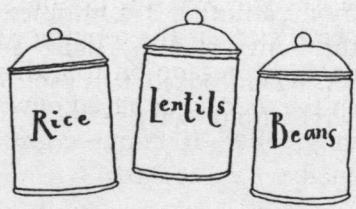

Stir-fry – stir crazy

Stir-fries are so easy to make that teenagers can make their own. This age group will also enjoy Salmon Stir-fry (page 175) or Almond Tofu Stir-fry (page 176).

Immune-boosting Chicken Stir-fry

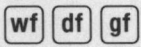

This is a really good one to start off with. You can cut up all the vegetables freshly yourself, or once in a while, for a super-speedy stir-fry, you can use the ready sliced ones from supermarkets.

SERVES 4 ADULTS

1 onion, peeled and thinly sliced
2.5 cm (1 inch) cube fresh ginger, thinly sliced
1 clove garlic, peeled and chopped
1 tablespoon extra-virgin olive oil
450 g (1 lb) skinless, boneless chicken breasts, cut into thin strips
sliced vegetables including peppers, pak choi, carrots, bean
    sprouts, mangetout and baby corn *or* 1 × 300 g pack of stir-fry
    vegetables and 1 × 300 g pack of bean sprouts
1 tablespoon tamari soy sauce
1 tablespoon raw runny honey
a handful chopped fresh coriander

Stir-fry the onion, ginger and garlic in the olive oil. Add the chicken and stir-fry for a further 3–4 minutes. Add the mixed vegetables with the honey and soy sauce and stir-fry for a further 4–5 minutes. When cooked, toss some chopped coriander over the top. Serve with brown rice.

Alternatives

Replace the chicken with either of the following:

- Cashew nuts – roast under the grill and toss in at the end
- Duck breast – use skinless, boneless breasts

Other delicious healthy main courses

Panna

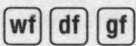

My mother gave me this recipe, which contains all the vital nutrients needed by this age group. As a teenager I loved it, so I hope yours do too.

SERVES 4 ADULTS

1 onion, peeled and chopped
1 tablespoon extra-virgin olive oil
1 packet fresh baby leaf spinach
a sprig tarragon
a handful parsley
2 hard-boiled organic eggs
1 tin sardines in oil
½ small tin anchovies

In a pan, cook the onion in the olive oil until transparent. Add the spinach, tarragon and parsley and continue cooking until the spinach has wilted. Put the hard-boiled eggs, sardines, anchovy fillets and spinach mixture into the food processor, and whizz until smooth. Put in the fridge for a couple of hours and serve with fresh bread, crackers or crudités.

Seafood Paella

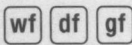

I was recently given a paella pan and I am now hooked. They are so easy to make and can feed hundreds of hungry teenagers! This recipe is particularly good for the immune system, as it is packed full of antioxidants and essential fatty acids. A bonus is that the leftovers will keep until the next day.

SERVES 4 ADULTS

1 onion, peeled and finely chopped
2 cloves garlic, peeled and crushed
1 red pepper, deseeded and diced
1 green pepper, deseeded and diced
2 tablespoons extra-virgin olive oil
a pinch turmeric
2 handfuls calamari (squid) rings
2 handfuls peeled prawns
1 handful fresh cockles or similar shellfish (without the shells)
2 plum tomatoes, skinned and chopped
375 g (12 oz) long grain brown rice or paella rice
900 ml (1½ pints) stock made from low-salt Marigold Swiss
    vegetable bouillon powder
1 cup frozen peas
a handful chopped parsley

In a paella pan or large flat frying pan, gently cook the onion, garlic and peppers in the olive oil until soft. Add the turmeric and cook for 1 minute. Add the squid, prawns and cockles and stir for a couple of minutes. Add the tomatoes along with the rice. Cook for 2 minutes. Add the stock and peas. Raise the heat and allow the pan to bubble very hard for a couple of minutes. Stir well, then leave to simmer gently for 25 minutes until all the stock has been absorbed. Sprinkle the chopped parsley on top and serve direct from the pan with a large mixed salad.

Store Cupboard Paella

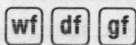

Another quick and easy recipe full of antioxidant nutrients.

SERVES 4 ADULTS

1 onion, peeled and finely chopped
2 cloves garlic, peeled and crushed
1 red pepper, deseeded and diced
1 green pepper, deseeded and diced
2 tablespoons extra-virgin olive oil
a pinch turmeric
2 skinless, boneless chicken breasts, cubed
½ cup bacon pieces (optional), cubed
3 handfuls peeled, cooked, frozen prawns (defrosted)
1 cup frozen peas
1 × 200 g tin sweetcorn (no sugar, no salt variety)
2 tablespoons tomato purée
375 g (12 oz) long grain brown rice or paella rice
900 ml (1½ pints) stock made from low-salt Marigold Swiss
   vegetable bouillon powder
a large handful chopped flat leaf parsley

In a paella pan or large flat frying pan, gently cook the onion, garlic and peppers in the olive oil until soft. Add the turmeric and cook for 1 minute. Add the bacon pieces and chicken and stir-fry for 10 minutes until cooked and golden brown. Add all the rest of the ingredients, stir well. Bring to the boil and allow to simmer for 25–30 minutes until all the stock has been absorbed. Sprinkle with the chopped parsley.

Bouillabaisse*

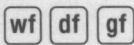

This recipe is packed full of zinc, iron and essential fatty acids. It is marvellous when you have a lot of people to feed as it can be doubled or tripled in quantity and can easily be thrown together in the morning to serve in the evening. It will also keep for a couple of days in the fridge.

SERVES 4 ADULTS

1 onion, peeled and chopped
1 clove garlic, peeled and crushed
1 tablespoon extra-virgin olive oil
450 g (1 lb) mixed fish and seafood (e.g. cod, wild salmon, fresh mackerel fillets, scallops, clams, prawns)
250 ml (9 fl oz) stock made from low-salt Marigold Swiss vegetable bouillon powder
2 tablespoons white wine
1 heaped tablespoon tomato purée
2 ripe tomatoes, skinned and chopped
a sprig rosemary
a sprig thyme
a handful chopped parsley

In a heavy pan, gently cook the onion and garlic in the olive oil until transparent. Cut the fish and seafood into bite-sized pieces as appropriate (i.e. leave prawns whole), add to the pan and cook gently for another 5 minutes. Add the stock, wine, tomato purée, tomatoes, rosemary and thyme. Bring to the boil and then simmer gently for 25 minutes. Sprinkle with parsley and serve with mashed potato or hunks of freshly baked bread and a green vegetable or salad.

Prawn Curry

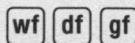

My mother gave me this recipe, and it really is delicious. It is best made with fresh tiger prawns, but the frozen ones are a good standby. You can choose whether or not to include the chilli, depending on your family's preference. Chillis help to shift mucus from the lungs and are therefore very useful when there are chest infections around. This is another recipe that you can make well in advance – just add the creamed coconut when you heat it to serve.

SERVES 4 ADULTS

2 medium onions, peeled and chopped
2 tablespoons extra-virgin olive oil
½ teaspoon chilli powder (optional)
½ teaspoon turmeric
1 teaspoon ground coriander
4 cloves
5 cm (2 inch) piece of cinnamon stick
2 teaspoons grated ginger
3 bay leaves
4 tomatoes, skinned and chopped
1 teaspoon raw honey
450 g (1 lb) large fresh *or* frozen cooked tiger prawns (defrosted)
5 cm (2 inch) cube creamed coconut

Gently sauté the onions in the olive oil. Add the spices and bay leaves and cook for a couple of minutes, stirring all the time. Add the tomatoes along with the honey. Bring the pan to simmering point. Add the prawns and gently simmer for 5 minutes. Just before serving remove the bay leaves, cloves and cinnamon stick, add the creamed coconut and stir until dissolved. Serve with brown rice, a mixture of chutneys and an oriental vegetable such as pak choi or mustard tops.

Mega Salads

These are a perfect lunch for a health- and weight-conscious teenager. You can make them meals in themselves.

    an iceberg lettuce
    a packet green leaf lettuce (e.g. rocket, watercress, baby cos,
        lollo rosso)
    1 red pepper
    1 yellow pepper
    radishes
    grated fennel
    chicory leaves
    sweetcorn kernels (no sugar, no salt variety)
    tinned pulses (no sugar, no salt variety)
    toasted sunflower, pumpkin and sesame seeds
    roasted cashew nuts
    fresh griddled tuna fish chunks
    hard-boiled organic egg halves
    leftover roast chicken slices
    smoked trout slices
    fresh olives
    sun-dried tomatoes
    cubes of cheddar *or* feta *or* soya *or* goat's cheese
    raisins
    grated carrot
    cooked green beans or mangetout or sugar snaps

Salad Dressing 1

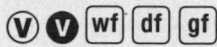

A lovely, clean, refreshing Mediterranean dressing.

SERVES 4 ADULTS

2 tablespoons good-quality balsamic vinegar
3–4 tablespoons extra-virgin olive oil
1 tablespoon chopped basil *or* fresh coriander

Whisk up all the ingredients together and pour over a salad.

Salad Dressing 2

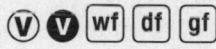

This classic dressing will be enjoyed by all ages. Its keeping qualities vary (see below).

SERVES 4 ADULTS

1 small clove garlic, peeled and crushed
1 dessertspoon Dijon mustard
1 dessertspoon raw runny honey
3 tablespoons apple cider vinegar
6 tablespoons extra-virgin olive oil (*or* flaxseed oil if being eaten straightaway)

Combine the garlic with the mustard and honey to form a paste. Slowly add the cider vinegar, mixing until you get a smooth sauce. Add the oil, mixing thoroughly. If you have used olive oil you can keep the dressing in the fridge, where it will thicken further. However, though flaxseed oil and cold-pressed sunflower seed oil are excellent oils for all the family, they do not keep well, and dressing made from them cannot be stored in this way.

Salad Dressing 3

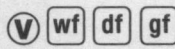 Ⓥ wf df gf

A delicious mayonnaise for coleslaws and chunky salads.

SERVES 4 ADULTS

1 clove garlic, peeled
1 organic egg
1 heaped teaspoon English mustard powder
juice of a lemon
150 ml (¼ pint) extra-virgin olive oil
black pepper

Put the garlic, egg, mustard powder and lemon juice in the food processor and whizz until smooth. While the blade is still running, pour the olive oil very slowly through the funnel until you have a smooth mayonnaise. Add a little more olive oil if necessary for desired consistency, and season to taste with black pepper.

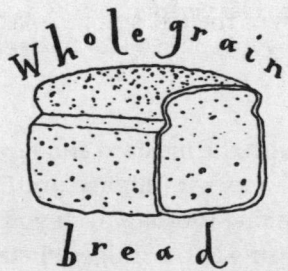

Goat's Cheese Salad

This is a great light lunch for those with cow's milk allergy. It also makes a delicious starter for a dinner party. You can make it well in advance.

SERVES 4 ADULTS

8 thick slices wholemeal bread
400 g (12 oz) chevre blanc (goat's cheese)
2 red peppers, deseeded and cut in half
1 clove garlic, cut in half
green salad leaves
red onion, peeled and thinly sliced
good-quality balsamic vinegar

Preheat the oven to 190°C/375°C/gas 5. Using a pastry cutter, cut out a round from each piece of bread. Thinly slice the goat's cheese. Bake the peppers, skin side up, for 30 minutes until the skins are darkening and the peppers are soft. Place on one side to cool. Lightly toast the bread. Rub the garlic halves over the toast rounds. Place a slice of cheese on top of each toast round and grill for a couple of minutes to melt the cheese. Arrange the salad leaves on 4 plates and place 2 cheese toasts on top of each. Skin the peppers, cut into slivers and arrange on the plates along with thin slices of the red onion. Splash on some balsamic vinegar.

Corn Tortillas with Mixed Beans and Vegetables

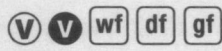

These are my most recent discovery. Unlike shop-bought tortillas, they are wheat-free and not filled with preservatives and other additives to increase their shelf life. They are surprisingly easy to make, too. Corn tortilla flour is available from some supermarkets.

SERVES 4 ADULTS

250 g (8 oz) corn tortilla flour
330 ml (½ pint) warm water

Mix the flour with the water in a bowl to form a dough. Mould into a ball and leave for a few minutes. Break the dough into 10 pieces. Roll each one into a ball. Using two pieces of clingfilm, with a dough ball in the middle, flatten it with a rolling pin, to form a very thin tortilla 'sandwich'. Carefully peel off the top sheet of clingfilm and turn the tortilla plus the remaining sheet of clingfilm upside down on your hand. Peel off the other clingfilm sheet and you will be left with the tortilla in the palm of your hand. In a very hot dry frying pan, cook the tortilla until the sides begin to shrink and dry out. Flip the tortilla over and cook for a further ½ minute. Place on a warm, clean drying up cloth while you cook the rest.

For the bean mash
1 tin mixed pulses, drained and rinsed
1 clove garlic, peeled
a handful coriander
¼–½ cup extra-virgin olive oil

Put all the ingredients apart from the olive oil in a food processor and mix well. Drizzle the olive oil through the top so that you only use what you think you will need.

For the vegetables
1 red onion
1 red pepper
1 yellow pepper
1 green pepper
1 tablespoon extra-virgin olive oil

Slice all the vegetables and fry in the oil for 15 minutes.

Tortilla serving suggestion

Once you have assembled all your ingredients, spread some bean mash on to the tortilla, add vegetables and maybe a slice of Thai Roast Chicken, roll up and eat straightaway.

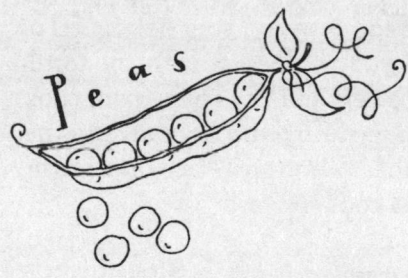

Thai Roast Chicken

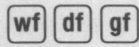

This roast chicken with a difference contains plenty of herbs and spices to keep your children well.

SERVES 4 ADULTS

1 whole chicken about 1.4 kg (3 lb) in weight
4 cloves garlic, peeled
a handful fresh coriander
2 tablespoons white wine
2 tablespoons coconut milk
1 tablespoon Thai fish sauce
1 teaspoon grated fresh ginger
2 tablespoons tamari soy sauce
black pepper

Preheat the oven to 220°C/425°F/gas 7. Mix all the ingredients except the chicken in a food processor. Place the chicken in a roasting dish and rub this marinade all over, pouring the excess inside the chicken. Cover with foil and roast for one hour, removing the foil after 40 minutes and basting the chicken with the liquid.

Thai Chicken Curry and Rice

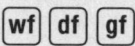

This wonderfully quick curry can feed an army in minutes. It is best made with the yellow curry paste available from Thai supermarkets (see Resources). If your teenagers don't like spicy food, reduce the amount of this paste. Thai fish sauce is available at most supermarkets.

SERVES 4 ADULTS

1 onion, peeled and chopped
2 cloves garlic, peeled and crushed
2 tablespoons extra-virgin olive oil
4 skinless, boneless chicken breasts, sliced
3 cups coconut milk
2 tablespoons yellow curry paste
4 tablespoons Thai fish sauce
1 tablespoon raw runny honey

Heat the oil in a large saucepan or wok and gently cook the onion and garlic until transparent. Slice the chicken, add and cook for 5–10 minutes. Add the rest of the ingredients and bring to the boil. Simmer for 5 minutes until the chicken is cooked through. Serve with brown rice and a green vegetable such as pak choi or Chinese cabbage.

Peanut Satay Spring Rolls

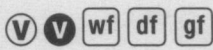

A vegetarian alternative that can be enjoyed by everyone, meat-eaters included. You will need 16 circles of rice paper.

MAKES 16

2 medium carrots, peeled and grated
150 g (5 oz) bean sprouts (½ a supermarket packet)
2 spring onions, thinly sliced
2 tablespoons smooth peanut butter
1 tablespoon tamari soy sauce

Preheat the oven to 220°C/425°F/gas 7. In a bowl mix the grated carrot, bean sprouts and spring onions with the peanut butter and soy sauce. Dip the rice paper sheets in warm water to soften them. Lay one by one on a plate, and place a dessertspoon of the bean sprout mixture in the middle. Roll up, folding the ends over, and place on a well-oiled baking tray. Brush with a little olive oil. Repeat with the rest of the spring rolls. Bake for 15–20 minutes until the spring rolls are cooked and firm to the touch.

Turkey Spring Rolls

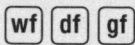

These wheat-free spring rolls are a triumph and so easy to make – all the family will enjoy helping. Turkey is a low-fat meat and therefore a much better choice than the minced pork which is commonly used in spring rolls. You will need 24 round sheets of rice paper, available from oriental supermarkets – make sure you choose the dried-wheat-free variety.

MAKES 24

1 clove garlic, peeled and crushed
1 tablespoon extra-virgin olive oil
250 g (9 oz) minced turkey
150 g (5 oz) bean sprouts (½ a supermarket packet)
150 g (5 oz) mixed stir-fry vegetables (½ a supermarket packet)
1 tablespoon tamari soy sauce

Preheat the oven to 220°C/425°F/gas 7. Heat the oil in a wok and cook the garlic for 1 minute. When the pan is really hot, add the turkey and stir-fry for a couple of minutes. Add the vegetables and cook for a further 2–3 minutes. Add the soy sauce and put to one side. Put the sheets of rice paper in warm water to soften them. Transfer them to a flat plate and place a dessertspoon of the turkey stir-fry in the middle of each. Add a couple more drops of soy sauce and roll up, folding over the ends last. Place the rolls on a well-oiled flat baking sheet and brush them lightly with olive oil. Bake for 10–15 minutes, until crunchy.

Baked Duck with Honey and Mustard Marinade

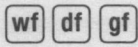 wf df gf

Duck contains three times as much iron as chicken, so it is an excellent choice of meat for teenagers who require lots of iron for growth and immune protection. It can, however, be very fatty, so either buy skinned breasts or remove the skin yourself before or after cooking.

SERVES 4 ADULTS

1 tablespoon wholegrain mustard
1 tablespoon raw runny honey
4 duck breasts, skinned

Preheat the oven to 220°C/425°F/gas 7. Make a marinade by combining the mustard and honey, and cover the duck breasts in it. Lay out on an oiled roasting pan, cover and bake for 20 minutes or until cooked through. Let the duck sit for 5 minutes before serving. Serve with sweet potato chips and a large green salad.

Mediterranean Chicken Casserole

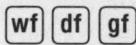

This, I think, is my favourite recipe in the whole book. It was simply by accident that I liquidised the gravy in the first place, but the result was pure nectar. Because it is full of immune-boosting phytonutrients, this one is an absolute winner on all counts.

SERVES 4 ADULTS

1 onion, peeled and sliced
1 clove garlic, peeled and crushed
1 red pepper, deseeded and sliced into strips
1 yellow pepper, deseeded and sliced into strips
2 tablespoons extra-virgin olive oil
1 chicken
a handful black pitted olives
20 cherry tomatoes
a sprig thyme
150 ml (¼ pint) stock made from low-salt Marigold Swiss
   vegetable bouillon powder

Preheat the oven to 220°C/425°F/gas 7. In a heavy casserole pan cook the onions, garlic and the peppers in the olive oil until the onion goes transparent. Add the chicken and surround it with the other ingredients. Put the lid on the casserole and bake for about an hour, until the chicken is cooked through. Transfer the chicken to a serving dish with high sides. Scoop out a generous portion of vegetables and place on top of the chicken. Skim any fat off the sauce and transfer the remainder to a liquidiser or food processor. Whizz it up and pour it around the chicken.

Immune-boosting Venison*

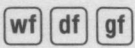

This wheat-free casserole is delicious and full of immune-boosting herbs.

SERVES 4 ADULTS

4 shallots, peeled and chopped

1 clove garlic, peeled and crushed

1 tablespoon extra-virgin olive oil

450 g (1 lb) diced venison

a generous splash red wine

5 fresh dates, pitted and chopped

600 ml (1 pint) stock made from low-salt Marigold Swiss vegetable bouillon powder

8 shiitake mushrooms, sliced

a sprig thyme

a handful chopped parsley for garnishing

Preheat the oven to 230°C/450°F/gas 8. In a heavy casserole pan, lightly cook the garlic and shallots with the olive oil. Add the meat, brown well, add the rest of the ingredients, bring to the boil, then transfer to the oven for 1 hour. You may need to add a little more stock if it cooks very quickly, so check the liquid level from time to time. When cooked, garnish with the parsley and serve with mashed potato and broccoli.

Baking and puddings

Nut and Seed Bread

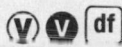

Rich in essential fatty acids and salt-free, this is an excellent bread to make for any age group. Serve with a variety of salads for a perfect Saturday family lunch.

SERVES 4 ADULTS

1 large onion, peeled and chopped
4 tablespoons extra-virgin olive oil
50 g (2 oz) pine nuts
450 g (1 lb) stoneground wholemeal flour or spelt flour
75 g (3 oz) chopped walnuts
75 q (3 oz) sesame seeds
2 teaspoons cumin seeds
2 teaspoons coriander seeds
a handful chopped fresh coriander
300 ml (½ pint) filtered water
1 packet easy-blend yeast

Gently fry the onion in a little of the oil for a couple of minutes. Add the pine nuts and allow to brown slightly. Put the flour, the walnuts and sesame seeds, the pine nuts and the onion in a large mixing bowl. Crush the cumin and coriander seeds in a pestle and mortar and add these as well. Stir in the chopped fresh coriander. Make a well in the centre of the mixture, pour in the water and sprinkle the yeast into the water. Mix the flour into the water and yeast and then add the olive oil to form a dough. Turn out on to a lightly floured surface and knead for 5 minutes. Put back in the bowl and cover with a damp, clean drying up cloth. Leave in a warm place for an hour to rise (not absolutely necessary if you are in a hurry – it will still taste jolly good!). Preheat the oven to 200°C/400°F/gas 6. Transfer the dough to a lightly oiled cake tin or baking tray. Sprinkle with a few extra sesame seeds and pine nuts and bake for 40 minutes. Turn the bread out on to a rack and leave to cool.

Yeast-free Bread

SERVES 4 ADULTS

450 g (1 lb) stoneground wholemeal flour or spelt flour
2 teaspoons bicarbonate of soda
25 g (1 oz) butter or unhydrogenated margarine
300 ml (10 fl oz) buttermilk *or* natural yoghurt

Preheat the oven to 200°C/400°F/gas 6. Mix all the ingredients together in a food processor to form a dough. Turn on to a lightly floured surface and knead into a round loaf. Place on a baking tray and cut a cross in the top. Bake for 30 minutes until it has risen and is golden brown and crusty on the top. It can be eaten warm, or cooled on a wire rack. Eat the same day as bread, or it will toast very well the next day.

Baked Fruit and Proper Custard

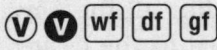

So simple, but another way of serving fruit with the addition of molasses, rich in trace elements and therefore good for the immune system. Instead of custard, you could cover the baked fruit with Nutty Crumble (page 158).

SERVES 4 ADULTS

1 organic apple, cored and sliced
1 organic pear, cored and sliced
1 organic nectarine, stoned and sliced
a handful raisins
⅓ cup warmed apple juice
1 tablespoon blackstrap molasses

Preheat the oven to 180°C/350°F/gas 4. Lay out the sliced fruit in a greased ovenware dish, sprinkle the raisins on top and pour over the apple juice with the molasses mixed in well. Bake in the oven for 30 minutes, until the fruit is soft and the apple juice is reduced and sticky. Serve with Proper Custard (below).

Proper Custard

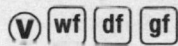

SERVES 4 ADULTS

2 organic egg yolks
1 heaped teaspoon cornflour
1 teaspoon vanilla extract
300 ml (½ pint) soya milk or semi-skimmed milk
1 tablespoon maple syrup (optional)

In a 600 ml (1 pint) jug, mix the egg yolks with the cornflour and vanilla extract. Warm the milk in a saucepan. Just before it reaches boiling point, pour the milk into the jug and mix well. Pour the mixture back into the pan and, stirring all the time, simmer gently until the custard has thickened to the desired consistency.

Drinks

Blackcurrant and Apple Juice Smoothie

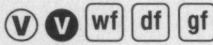

SERVES 4 ADULTS

1 frozen banana (page 153)
1 tablespoon tinned blackcurrants in apple juice
1 cup apple juice
1 teaspoon of an oil blend (see Resources)

Combine all the ingredients in a liquidizer or Magimix and blend until smooth. If you want a fruit fool for a pudding, just omit the apple juice. All young children will enjoy drinking this, especially if it comes with a straw!

Tropical Smoothie

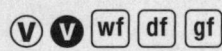

SERVES 4 ADULTS

2 frozen bananas (page 153)
½ cup pineapple chunks
½ cup coconut milk

Whizz up all the ingredients in a food processor or liquidiser. Serve in a cup with a straw.

Banana Berry Smoothie

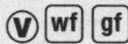

SERVES 4 ADULTS

2 bananas
¼ cup apple juice
½ cup natural yoghurt or silken tofu
½ cup frozen berries

Whizz up all the ingredients in a food processor or liquidiser
and serve in a cup with a straw.

Healthy alternatives to soft drinks

- Water
- Appletise
- Aqua Libra
- Meridian blackcurrant and apple
  concentrate, diluted (available from healthfood shops)
- Freshly squeezed juices, slightly diluted with water
- Freshly squeezed vegetable juice
  cocktail
- V8 vegetable juice (available in cans or bottles from super-
  markets)
- Fruit smoothies

Weekly Menu Suggestions

	Breakfast	Lunch	Tea
MONDAY	Liquid Energy Breakfast (page 196) Diluted juice or appropriate milk	Packed lunch or school lunch	Family Macaroni Cheese (page 205) Tropical Smoothie (page 232) Water or freshly squeezed juice to drink
TUESDAY	Fruitful (page 197) Diluted juice or appropriate milk	Packed lunch or school lunch	Seafood Paella (page 212) Fresh fruit and Flapjacks (page 184) Water or freshly squeezed juice to drink
WEDNESDAY	Organic muesli Diluted juice or appropriate milk	Packed lunch or school lunch	Thai Chicken Curry and Rice (page 223) and pak choi Melon slices and Honey Cakes (page 185) Water or Aqua Libra
THURSDAY	Pumpkin Seed Porridge (page 198) Diluted juice or appropriate milk	Packed lunch or school lunch	Immune-boosting Venison (page 228) and broccoli Fresh fruit and yoghurt Water or Appletise
FRIDAY	Instant Energy Fruit Smoothie (page 197) Diluted juice or appropriate milk	Packed lunch or school lunch	Corn Tortillas with Mixed Beans and Vegetables (page 220) Fruit and Banana Yoghurt Cake (page 187) Water or freshly squeezed juice to drink
SATURDAY	Muesli Bars (page 163) Diluted juice or appropriate milk	Vegetable soup Fruit	Turkey Spring Rolls (page 225) Baked Fruit and Proper Custard (page 230–231) Water or freshly squeezed juice to drink
SUNDAY	Scrambled eggs on toast Diluted juice or appropriate milk	Thai Roast Chicken (page 222) and vegetables Blackberry and apple crumble and cream	Sandwich platter with cucumber and carrot stick and popcorn Banana Berry Smoothie (page 233) Water or V8 vegetable juice to drink

PART THREE

•

Treating Infections Naturally

This section explains the best natural
treatments for dealing with common
childhood illnesses. Getting ill is an
important part of your child's immune
development and the following advice
will enable you to give her immune
system the support it needs.

Chapter 13

•

FIGHTING DISEASES NATURALLY

CHILDREN DO GET ILL. It is an important part of their immune development. But more often than not their illnesses are short-lived and serve merely to prime their immune systems and strengthen their defences. While this is happening it is important to support their immune systems and allow their bodies the time and space to heal themselves. Obviously there are times when medical intervention is important, and in some cases the diseases can be life-threatening, but this is rare. The most common illnesses your children are likely to encounter are viruses that cause colds and flu, sore throats, bacterial infections of the ear and chest, and common childhood diseases such as chicken pox and measles.

Have faith in your instincts as a parent

Dr Robert Mendelsohn, an American paediatrician and author of numerous books including *How to Raise a Healthy Child in Spite of Your Doctor,* has some very sound advice. I have found his work extremely instructive and comforting whilst raising my three children. Here are some of his beliefs:

- Most things get better by morning

- Parents and grandparents are wiser than doctors

- If your child doesn't feel sick, look sick and act sick, he probably isn't sick

- Give Mother Nature ample time to work her magic before you expose your child to the doctor

- Common sense is the most useful tool in dealing with illness. Your doctor is less likely to employ it than you are, and certainly no more able.

My own three children have been ill. I have had countless sleepless nights, and spent many a worrying hour going through the 'what ifs'! However, I am proud to say that none of them has ever had oral antibiotics; I am convinced that this is due mainly to their diet, but also partly to my trusting my instinct when I really needed to. I use plenty of support: I have a homeopath I can see when I need to, a naturopathic doctor who is on the end of a telephone in real emergencies, and I also visit our local doctor when I need a diagnosis. Trusting your maternal instincts when your children are ill takes practice, but when you have done it once it comes more naturally each time.

The healing power of a fever

When your child gets a fever, it can be very worrying. It is not, however, as most parents believe, something that needs to be suppressed the moment it arrives. Fever is an indication that your child is trying to burn off something which is not meant to be there. It is an extremely clever natural mechanism that the body employs to defend itself against unwanted pathogens.

The most common cause of fever is an infection by a virus or by bacteria. As the immune army gets to work to destroy whatever intruder they have identified in your child's body, chemicals called pyrogens get released. These are designed to raise the body temperature and make the cleansing exercise more efficient. The fever they produce is very beneficial. High body temperature stimulates the immune system to produce more white blood cells. It also increases the heart rate, so that white blood cells get delivered to the sites of infection more rapidly and their secretions are increased. In addition, heat increases antibody production and intensifies the effect of interferon (see page 7). It can also speed up chemical reactions, which may help body cells to repair themselves during a disease.

I find it rather comforting to think that a child's body works so hard to heal itself, and I would encourage any parent to think twice before reaching for the Calpol. Such medicines not only reduce the temperature and therefore the child's immune activity, but also mask the symptoms so that the child temporarily feels better. I think this is a real mistake, because the child is then likely to be doing things that will not be remotely helpful to the healing process – such as running around and eating. Whenever my children are ill I pop them into bed (usually mine) with a big jug of diluted organic apple juice and vitamin C and let them sleep, watch videos, read stories and get better. This normally does the trick beautifully and they recover incredibly quickly. Suppressing their symptoms through drugs can often lead to lingering illness.

Obviously fever has its beneficial limit – a raised temperature is different from a temperature spiralling out of control. It is also very important to look for other symptoms, such as rashes, difficulty in breathing or unnatural floppiness, which may indicate something more serious. But on the whole a raised temperature should not be an instant cause for alarm.

Treating a fever naturally

When your child has a temperature, here are some helpful hints on treating it naturally.

- The most important thing is to make sure that she does not get dehydrated, since the sweating and runny nose that often accompany a fever can deplete her body of fluids. Give your child a cup of tepid diluted apple juice (or blackcurrant and apple juice) every hour, and if she is a reluctant drinker pop a straw in, which will encourage her.

- If your child is not hungry, don't insist that she eats. Energy taken up digesting food is energy channelled away from the healing process, which requires a great deal. Make plenty of fresh raw juices (see juice boost recipes on page 244). Juices rehydrate your child's body, supply plenty of antioxidants and encourage the elimination of unwanted toxins. Most children love fresh raw juices, and these are all that is needed to see them through acute illness.

- Tepid sponging can be very effective at bringing down a fever naturally. However, some children don't like it, especially if they are in the shivery stage of a fever. For these children (and adults for that matter), a tummy compress can be an effective fever controller and detoxifier. Rip open the sides of an old cotton pillowcase (it must be cotton). It must be large enough to reach from under your child's armpit to her hips. Dip it in cold water and wring it out. Wrap it around her middle very quickly at least once, and fasten it with a nappy pin. On top wrap a thick, dry towel and fasten with another nappy pin. Pop some pyjama bottoms and some thick socks on the child and put her into bed. The important thing is not to let her get cold. You can take the compress off after half an hour, or, if she falls asleep with it on,

continues ▶

you can wait until morning. If your child is resistant to the above strategies, don't insist. Just keep her nice and cool and wipe her forehead with a cool flannel when needed. Children often know exactly what their body needs.

• If you are registered with a homeopath locally, they may recommend Belladona to reduce a fever. I find homeopathy is fantastic for treating childhood complaints, as children seem to respond so quickly and it is completely natural. To find a homeopath near you, see Resources.

Symptoms of meningitis

The symptoms of meningitis often come on very quickly and call for very prompt action. The disease involves a combination of some of the symptoms below. If you are ever unsure, always act. Prompt treatment can mean the difference between life and death.

- Purple rash
- Fever
- Headache, often severe
- Aversion to bright lights
- Vomiting
- Stiff neck and back
- Drowsiness and confusion

In a baby, look for the following:

- Purple rash, sometimes only pinprick size, which does not fade when a glass in pressed against it
- Fever
- A high-pitched cry

- A bulging fontanelle
- Aversion to bright lights
- Fits or loss of consciousness

Ten steps for dealing with colds and viruses

You will encounter endless colds and other viruses through your child's life. These escalate when they start school and then seem to taper off once the child is over the age of eight.

1. At the first sign of a sniffle, mix 300 ml (½ pint) of fresh apple juice with 300 ml (½ pint) filtered water and add 1,000 mg of powdered vitamin C. Offer it at regular intervals through the day, until the whole jug has been drunk. For a baby under one, use vitamin C drops instead (see Resources).

2. Give your children a juice boost (see page 244) packed full of immune-boosting nutrients and antioxidants.

3. Zinc lozenges can be very useful for boosting the immune system, combating colds and soothing a sore throat. Zinc drops are available for babies (see Resources). Follow for three days the appropriate therapeutic dosage for your child's age.

4. Avoid mucous-forming foods which have a tendency to increase and thicken mucus. These foods are milk, cream, cheese, yoghurt, eggs, meat and sugary foods. If your child gets really thick colds, with a heavy mucus which makes it difficult for her to breathe and gives her a rattly cough, you can use a homeopathic mucous-dissolver. This is very effective on babies as well (see Resources).

5. Avoid fatty foods, which thicken lymph and encourage a sluggish lymphatic system. Drinking lots of fluid helps to thin mucus and prevent a sluggish lymphatic system.

6. Avoid sugary foods, which apart from forming mucus suppress your child's immune system. Use raw honey or tea tree honey medicinally (see Hot Toddy, page 248).

7. Echinacea and goldenseal stimulate the immune system. Echinacea is both antibacterial and antiviral. Goldenseal is antibacterial and noted for healing irritated mucous membranes. There are various combinations on the market but the best, in my opinion, are available by mail order from Gaia's Children (see Resources).

8. Garlic has antibacterial properties and helps detoxify the body. Add it raw to your cooking whenever you can. A good way to disguise it for those who dislike the taste is in salad dressing (page 217).

9. Just before bed make up a Hot Toddy (see page 248). Ginger helps to increase sweating, which cleanses the body and reduces the strength of a cold.

10. Give your child elderberry extract, which research has shown to be antiviral and to reduce the length of a cold. You can now buy this extract in a children's formula (see Resources). Give it to them at the correct dosage for three days.

Mucous-formers and mucous-reducers

Foods that tend to increase mucus

- cow's milk, cream, cheese, yoghurt
- ice cream
- eggs
- sugary foods
- fried foods
- red meat
- too much salt
- rich foods

Foods that tend to reduce mucus

- garlic and onion
- celery
- citrus fruit
- parsley
- chicken broth
- watercress
- horeseradish
- green tea

What to do if your child has to take antibiotics

- Once the course of antibiotics is finished, give your child a pro-biotic supplement for one month (see Resources). Probiotic supplements replace the beneficial bacteria lost during antibi-otic use, preventing up to 50 per cent of infections that might otherwise have occurred after antibiotic use.

- Support her immune system by using the immune-boosting herbs echinacea and goldenseal (see Resources).

- Feed her plenty of antioxidant- and zinc-rich foods to strength-en her defences (see page 44–6).

- Avoid sugar, which suppresses her immune system and may make her more susceptible to reinfection.

The healing power of raw juices

Raw juices are not only delicious but also exceptionally rich in health-promoting enzymes as well as vitamins, minerals and trace elements, which are particularly helpful in restoring bio-chemical balance to the body. Europeans have traditionally used juice fasts as a way of reviving their bodies after the winter months. Juices are particularly good as part of an immune-boosting programme for your children and, because they taste so good, will not be met with much resistance.

The bore about juices is that only those made from citrus fruit can be made by hand or in a food processor, so a juicer is neces-sary (see Resources). Here are some recipes to get your family on the way to tip-top health.

Juice boosts

These make roughly 300 ml (½ pint) of juice depending on the size of the fruit and vegetables you are using. To prevent nutrient loss they should be drunk straightaway. It is, as ever, best to use organic fruit and vegetables, but this is not always possible. Juice boosts can be drunk every day or just when your child is showing cold or flu symptoms.

Carrot and Apple

This is a brilliant juice to start with. It is rich in vitamin C and beta-carotene and children will love the taste and its natural sweetness. This combination makes a great base for being more adventurous, for instance adding a handful of parsley or some beetroot.

> 3 organic carrots
> 3 organic eating apples

Top and tail and peel the carrots. Peel, core and chop the apples. Juice, and serve straightaway.

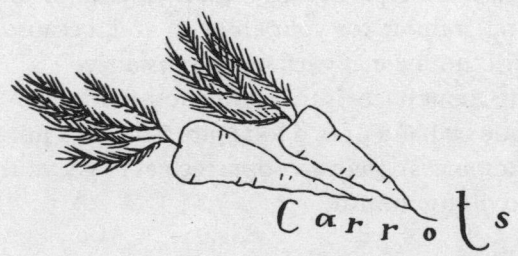

Cantaloupe Melon and Raspberry

Cantaloupe melon is rich in the potent antioxidant betacarotene. Raspberries, full of vitamin C, are traditionally used to cleanse and detoxify the digestive system as well as to soothe childhood illnesses and as a cooling remedy for a fever.

½ large cantaloupe melon
1 small punnet raspberries

Scoop out the flesh of the melon, and discard the seeds. Juice the raspberries first and then the melon. Serve straightaway.

Blackcurrant and Apple

This juice is also nice gently warmed and is very soothing to sore throats.

3 organic eating apples
a small tin blackcurrants in juice

Peel and core the apples. Juice with the blackcurrants and serve immediately.

Tonics

These tonics, as the juices above, make roughly 300 ml (½ pint) depending on the size of the vegetables. Tonics can be drunk at any time but are particularly good when your child is under par or appears tired.

Trace Element Tonic

This tonic is full of beta-carotene, vitamin C, potassium, iron and other trace elements from the molasses. It is great when your child seems worn out.

> ½ watermelon (including the seeds), cut into chunks
> 1 very ripe banana
> ½ teaspoon blackstrap molasses

Put the banana through the juicer first, then the watermelon, which will flush through the banana flesh. Once juiced, stir in the molasses. Don't be tempted into thinking more molasses is better – it is so strong that it will overpower the flavour of the juice if you overdo it.

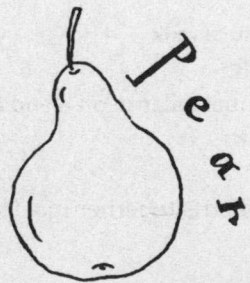

Antioxidant Tonic

This juice is packed full of antioxidant vitamins as well as phytonutrients: lycopene from the tomatoes, carotenoids from the carrots and allicin from the garlic, as well as plenty of potassium from the celery.

    4–5 organic carrots
    3–5 sticks organic celery
    1 small clove garlic, peeled
    2 ripe tomatoes
    a sprig of parsley

Juice all the ingredients together and serve straightaway.

Essential Fatty Acid Tonic

This is a great drink to mix in a food processor. It is a very good way of disguising essential fatty acids and can be served in a feeder cup for the very young or a beaker for older children. This tonic can be drunk every day and is a good one to give daily to your children if they are showing symptoms of essential fatty acid deficiency (see page 51).

    1 cup rice milk or soya milk
    2 very ripe bananas
    1 tablespoon Essential Balance oil blend (see Resources)
    a squeeze of lemon

Whizz all the ingredients together in a food processor, and serve straightaway.

Other juice goodies

Frozen Juice Lollies

These are a great source of vitamins, and are a wonderfully soothing remedy for sore throats.

MAKES 4 SMALL LOLLIES

4 organic eating apples

Peel, core and chop the fruit. Use more if you need to. Juice and pour into small lolly moulds. Freeze straightaway.

> **Variation**
> Peel and juice 4 organic oranges and 1 organic mango instead of the apples

Hot Toddy

When your child is unwell this is a wonderfully comforting drink to give at bedtime. It will soothe sore throats and contains useful antibacterial agents.

MAKES 1 SERVING

juice of ½ lemon
a thin slice root ginger
2 teaspoons manuka (tea tree) honey
enough warm boiled water to fill a beaker or mug

Squeeze the lemon into a cup or beaker, add the honey and ginger and fill with water.

Healing soups

The Very Best Immune-boosting Soup for All the Family

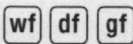

This is my favourite recipe for those evenings when you have been out with the family all day and are too tired to cook. It is also marvellous as an instant family meal at any time, incredibly quick to prepare and full of immune-boosting elements. You will have to adapt it to your children's age group. As it is a broth and quite difficult to negotiate, it probably suits the over-fives best!

THIS MAKES 1 ADULT BOWL

1 cluster of rice noodles
300 ml (½ pint) stock made from Marigold Swiss vegetable
 bouillon powder
1 clove garlic, peeled and crushed
a couple of slices leftover cooked chicken breast (optional)
1 thin slice root ginger, chopped
a handful chopped coriander or parsley

Place the rice noodles in a heatproof glass bowl, cover with freshly boiled water and soak for 5 minutes. Put the stock in a large soup bowl, add the garlic and the chicken slices, if using, and the ginger. Toss in the soaked rice noodles, and sprinkle with the herbs.

Immune-boosting Soup for the Under-fives (and the Rest of the Family)

SERVES 2 ADULTS AND 2 CHILDREN

1 onion, peeled and sliced
1 tablespoon extra-virgin olive oil
a handful shiitake mushrooms, washed and sliced
1 clove garlic, peeled and crushed
1 thin slice ginger
1.2 litres (2 pints) vegetable stock (see page 102)
3 large carrots, peeled and sliced
1 sweet potato, chopped
½ cup pearl barley
1 head broccoli
a handful chopped parsley

Gently cook the onions in the olive oil until transparent. Add the mushrooms, garlic and ginger, and cook for a further minute. Pour in the stock together with the carrots, sweet potato and barley and simmer for 40 minutes. Add the broccoli and simmer for a further 5–10 minutes. Remove the ginger and serve sprinkled with parsley. Liquidise to form a thick, hearty soup for younger children.

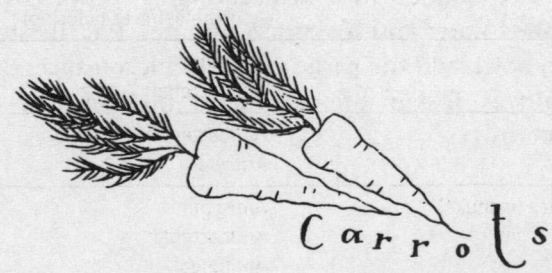

Carrots

Bug beaters

All these items are mentioned in the book, either in recipes or as part of recommended herbal products.

Basil	Antibacterial Antiparasitic
Blueberry leaf	Antibacterial Antiviral
Cranberry	Antibacterial (especially urinary tract infections)
Echinacea	Broad-spectrum immune enhancer Antibacterial Antifungal
Elderberry	Antiviral
Flavonoids (anthocyandins and proanthocyanidins)	Antibacterial Antiviral
Garlic	Antiseptic Antibacterial Antiviral Antifungal
Goldenseal	Antibacterial Antifungal Antiparasitic Broad-spectrum immune enhancer Antipyretic (fever-reducing)
Olive leaf	Antibacterial Antiviral Antifungal Antipyretic (fever-reducing)
Oregano	Antifungal Antibacterial
St John's wort	Antibacterial Antiviral
Tea tree honey (manuka)	Antiseptic Antibacterial Antifungal

Natural prescriptions – a quick A–Z

Condition	Remedies
Colds and flu	<ul><li>Juice boosts (see page 244)</li><li>Immune-boosting soups (see page 249–250)</li><li>Vitamin C and zinc</li><li>Elderberry extract (see Resources)</li><li>Avoid mucous-forming foods</li><li>VIR homeopathic drops (see Resources)</li></ul>
Colic	<ul><li>Fennel tea – a teabag dipped into a bottle of boiled water and offered to the baby</li><li>If breast-feeding, drink camomile and fennel tea which will be passed on to your baby through your breast milk</li></ul>
Constipation	<ul><li>Increase raw fruit and vegetables, especially carrots</li><li>Avoid refined foods and use wholegrains</li><li>Make sure your child is drinking enough water</li><li>Serve porridge for breakfast as a goodsource of fibre</li><li>Never use bran, which is too abrasive for a young digestive system</li></ul>
Conjunctivitis (sticky eye)	<ul><li>Bathe the eye three times a day with a solution made up of 300 ml (½ pint) boiled water, 1 teaspoon sea salt and 10 drops Euphrasia (eyebright formula). See the doctor if it doesn't clear up within 3 days</li><li>If you are breast-feeding, squeeze some breast milk into your infant's or child's eye. It contains natural antibacterial agents (see page 79) which are extremely effective at combating eye infections</li></ul>
Coughs	<ul><li>Juice boosts (see page 244) rich in beta-carotene, which soothe mucous membranes</li><li>Muc Liquescence (see Resources) if cough thick and rattly</li><li>Avoid mucous-forming foods</li></ul>
Diarrhoea	<ul><li>Give no food until the diarrhoea has stopped</li><li>Give plenty of liquid (water and very diluted fresh apple juice)</li><li>Rice milk is a traditional remedy for infant diarrhoea and is very effective for a baby as it is dairy-free, naturally sweet and non-mucous-forming.</li></ul>

Condition	Remedies
	• Use a probiotic supplement (see Resources) to replace the beneficial bacteria necessary for digestive health
Earache	• Avoid mucous-forming foods
	• Use hopi candles for children over five (see Resources)
	• Use herbal ear drops (see Resources)
	• Wrap a hot water bottle in a towel and place on the sore ear. This is very comforting
Fever	• Keep your child cool
	• Use homeopathic remedies where appropriate
	• Plenty of rest
	• Use paracetamol as a last resort
Sore throat	• Zinc and vitamin C lozenges
	• Herbal throat sprays (see Resources)
	• Avoid sugar
	• Juice boosts (page 244)
	• A teaspoon of manuka honey eaten slowly to coat the throat
	• Hot Toddy (see page 248)
Tummy aches	• Establish your child's bowel habits
	• Use a natural laxative such as fig syrup, if necessary, increase fruit and vegetable intake and add 1 tablespoon flaxseed oil to their daily diet
	• Have a cuddle – many tummy aches are emotional ones
	• Look for food allergies if your child gets recurrent tummy ache
	• If severe, always get the problem checked by a doctor
Vomiting	• Give no food for 24 hours
	• Give plenty of liquid, which should be sipped, to prevent dehydration
	• If vomiting accompanies diarrhoea, give a rehydration drink. You can buy these at chemists or make your own. Mix 1 teaspoon sea salt with 2 dessertspoons sugar, 1 litre (2 pints) water and 600 ml (1 pint) orange juice. Offer a glass of this mixture every hour after a bout of vomiting. Only allow your child to sip gently – drinking fast will just cause more vomiting

Should my child take nutritional supplements?

I am a firm believer that prevention is better than cure. Ensuring that your children have a healthy diet 100 per cent of the time is practically impossible, so I always recommend taking out insurance by giving them a really good-quality multivitamin and mineral each day. Using supplements designed for children will guarantee that you are not giving them too much of anything, and it will give them added protection against the effects of environmental pollution and those inevitable minor dietary indiscretions.

For babies over six months, you can use vitamin drops. Once over a year they can move on to a vitamin and mineral powder that can be added to food, and from two they can progress on to chewables (see Resources).

Using vitamins and minerals therapeutically during illness should be done with the advice of a nutritionist or doctor trained in nutritional therapy, but here is a guide to immune-boosting vitamins and minerals that can be used therapeutically when your children are ill. Don't use therapeutic amounts for longer than three days.

Three day Therapeutic Dosages

Vitamins and minerals	6–12 months	1–2 years	3–4 years	5–6 years	7–11 years	12–15 years	16–18 years
Beta-carotene	2,000iu	2,500iu	2,500iu	3,000iu	4,000iu	5,000iu	5,000iu
	One dose a day						
Vitamin C	60mg	150mg	200mg	200–500mg	250–500mg	250–500mg	250–500mg
	One dose, three times a day						
Zinc	6mg	10mg	10mg	10mg	10mg	10mg	10mg
	One dose a day						

Essential Fatty Acid Supplementation

FFA	Source	0–12 months	1–5 years	6–18 years
Omega-3 & Omega-6	Essential balance oil blend	–	1 tablespoon daily	2+ tablespoons daily
Omega-3	Fish oils	–	1 teaspoon daily	1 teaspoon to 1 tablespoon daily
Omega-3	Flaxseed oil	1 teaspoon daily	1 tablespoon daily	2+ tablespoons daily
Omega-6	Evening Primrose oil	1 x 500 mg capsule rubbed on tummy daily	up to 3 g daily for short-term treatment of eczema	up to 3 g daily for treatment of skin conditions

Your child is likely to only ever need one type of EFA supplementation, but this chart shows you which essential fatty acids are present in which oils. See Resources for suppliers.

Glossary

Allergen – Any substance that causes an allergy. It may, for example, be pollen that can trigger hay fever or peanuts that can cause anaphylactic shock.

Anaphylactic shock – A life threatening form of allergic reaction (in response to a food or insect sting) in which vast quantities of histamine are released throughout the body causing rapid swelling and breathing difficulty. Rapid medical treatment is required and this condition can be fatal.

Antibiotic – Drugs used to combat bacterial or fungal infections. Taken orally they can upset the balance of the intestinal bacteria resulting in digestive discomfort. Overuse is blamed for the current rising trend of antibiotic resistant bacteria. Antibiotics are not effective against viruses.

Antibody – Part of the immune army, capable of destroying bacteria and other potentially harmful substances. They are manufactured in the lymphoid tissue, such as the spleen, in response to an invader such as an allergen or a virus. They are transported around the body in the bloodstream. Each antibody combats a particular infection, for example, a chicken pox antibody would not fight a cold virus. Once the body has an effective antibody it becomes immune to that disease.

Antihistamine – Histamine is one of the substances released by the cells of the body in the case of allergy. Antihistamines are drugs that counteract the effects of histamine and are used in the treatment of hay fever, urticaria, rashes, insect bites and stings. Natural anti-histamines mentioned in this book are vitamin C and quercetin.

Antioxidants – Substances that detoxify free radicals. These include vitamins A, C, E, beta-carotene, zinc, selenium and many other non-essential substances such as bioflavanoids, lycopene, carotenoids, anthocyanidins and proanthocyanidins.

Atopy – Hereditary hypersensitivity which may cause familial hay fever, eczema, asthma or migrane.

Autoimmune disease – If the body does not recognise 'self' it goes into self-destruct mode and an immune assault is waged against body cells instead of a foregin invader Pernicious anaemia, rheumatoid arthritis and ulcerative colitis are all examples of auto-immune diseases.

Beta-carotene – The yellow-orange pigment that gives food – carrots, apricots, mangoes and cantaloupe melons – their bright colours. It is an antioxidant that can protect the body against free radicals. It can also be turned into vitamin A by the body as and when it needs it.

Bioflavonoid – Compounds found in fruits such as lemons, grapefruit, cherries, blackcurrants and buckwheat. Examples of bioflavonoids are hesperidin, rutin, and quercetin. With strong antioxidant properties these substances are thought to help prevent certain forms of cancer.

Carcinogen – Any substance that may produce cancer in living cells.

Coeliac disease – A condition found in childhood in which the small intestine is unable to absorb food properly. It is due to sensitivity to gluten, a protein found in certain grains such as wheat, barley and rye. Coeliacs have to follow a strict gluten-free diet to prevent damaging their small intestine.

Complex carbohydrates – A collective name for starches and fibre, which have a more complicated chemical structure than sugars (simple carbohydrates) and are the healthier option.

Dairy-free – A diet that avoids all products made from cow's milk e.g. milk, cheese, yoghurt and sometimes butter. Dairy products are mucous forming and some children with recurrent ear infections or chest infections may benefit from an elimination period.

Empty calories – A food that contains calories without any nutritional benefit e.g. refined, white sugar.

Elimination diet – A diet which, carried out under medical supervision, excludes all foods except a very few in an attempt to isolate food allergies or intolerances. Some doctors now provide in-patient treatment during the course of an elimination diet.

Endorphins – Natural painkillers and tranquillisers produced in the brain. They are released at times of severe mental stress or stenuous exercise. Chocolate is believed to boost the endorphin levels in the brain, which may be the explanation for the feel good factor felt by 'chocoholics'!

Enzyme – Proteins produced by cells to act as catalysts, helping to speed up biological processes. They help us digest our food as well as many other functions. Each enzyme has a different function. The enzyme delta-6-desaturase is needed – with the help of zinc, magnesium, vitamin B6 and biotin – to convert essential fatty acids into anti-inflammatory prostaglandins.

Free radical – An atom or group of atoms with one or more impaired electron. Free radicals are very damaging to DNA and proteins and to the fat in cell membranes where a free radical chain reaction can be started. Antioxidants such as vitamin E and C, selenium, zinc, copper and manganese usually neutralise these free radicals. However, if too many are produced they can cause degenerative diseases such as heart disease and cancer. Free radicals are created by smoking, pollution, radiation, frying or barbecuing food as well as normal body processes as a by product of combustion.

Gluten – The protein of wheat and other grains. Some people are sensitive to gluten as in Coeliac Disease and need to follow a strict gluten-free diet. The other grains that contain gluten or similar protein and therefore best avoided are oats, barley and rye.

GM foods – Genes are the building blocks of living organisms. They are passed from generation to generation and carry the information controlling that particular organism's characteristics. Scientists have now found a way of identifying individual genes and their functions and transplanting genes from one plant or animal to another. At the moment, over 3,000 genetically-engineered foods are being tested. The ones we hear most about are tomatoes, soya, and maize (corn). Organic foods are not allowed to be genetically modified and therefore are the obvious choice when avoiding GM foods.

Homeopathy – A system of practice that is based on the premise that diseases can be cured by giving substances that cause the same symptoms. It is believed that the more dilute these substances are made, the more powerful their effect. Constitutional homeopathy is based on the premise that there are patterns of symptoms, which make up different constitutional types and will therefore benefit those with that pattern of symptoms. Homeopathic 'nosodes' were formulated by Dr Constance Herring. These remedies were made from diseased tissue or bodily tissues. In 1838 he and his colleagues used a homeopathic preparation of infected sheep's spleen to cure anthrax, at one time an almost certainly fatal disease.

Lymph – The clear plasma like liquid found in lymph vessels.

Lymphocytes – White blood cells involved in the body's immune system. B-lymphocytes produce antibodies and are divided into plasma cells that secrets the immunoglobins (Ig) and memory cells that act when the event that stimulated antibody selection occurs. T-lymphocytes help to protect against virus infections and cancer and are divided into helper cells, suppressor cells, cytotoxic cells, memory cells and mediators or delayed hypersensitivity. There are also large granular lymphocytes. These are the killer cells and the natural killer cells.

Macronutrient – General term for those nutrients required by the body in relatively large amounts to produce energy, such as protein, fat and carbohydrate.

Micro-organism – An organism which is too small to see with the naked eye. Bacteria and viruses are both examples.

Mucous membranes – The moist inner surface that lines the mouth, nasal sinuses, stomach, intestines and many other parts of the body. It secretes mucus which acts as a protective barrier and lubricant, as well as a medium for carrying enzymes.

Organic – Food that is produced without the use of chemical fertilisers, pesticides or herbicides. Organic animals are given organic feed and are not routinely given antibiotics or any hormones and other growth promoters. Organic food is free from artificial additives. Organic food does not however mean sugar-free so be sure to check the labels.

Oxalates – Found in rhubarb leaves (poisonous leaves), rhubarb stalks, spinach, sorrel and some nuts. They can inhibit the body's absorption of calcium and iron.

Pathogen – A disease causing organism.

Phytates – Occur in grains and pulses. They bind with minerals such as calcium, iron and zinc, making them more difficult for the body to absorb. Execessive intakes of, for example, wheat bran, could inhibit the body's absorption of these minerals. Avoid giving bran to your children.

Phytonutrients – Also known as phytochemicals. They are not vital to life and therefore are not classified as nutrients, like vitamins, as our lives do not depend on them. These substances have health promoting qualities that protect us from diseases such as heart disease and cancer. Phytochemicals mentioned in this book are allium, anthocyanidins, bioflavonoids, capsicum, carotenoids, chlorophyll and curcumin.

Prostaglandins – Substances that act as regulators throughout the body. Essential fatty acids are converted into prostaglandins with the help of certain nutrient co-factors.

Protein – A macronutrient which is needed by every cell in the body for growth, maintenance and repair.

Refined Foods – White sugar, white flour and white rice are all examples of refined foods. All refining results in huge nutrient loss.

Saturated fat – The main type of fat in meat and dairy products, such as butter and cheese as well as palm oil and coconut oil. A high intake of saturated fat has been linked to an increased risk of heart disease.

Tempeh – Soya product made from fermented soya beans. You can buy tempeh fresh, frozen, dried or pre-cooked. Like tofu, tempeh can be steamed, baked, fried or grilled.

Thymus gland – The thymus gland lies a the root of the neck behind the breastbone. It grows from birth to puberty and then starts to diminish in size but remains active. Its main function is the formation of T-lymphocytes which are an essential part of the immune system.

Tofu – Soya bean curd. It is an excellent meat and dairy substitute, high in protein and low in fat. There are two types: firm and silken. Firm is good in stir fries, stews and salads and silken is better in shakes and smooth puddings.

Trace elements – Minerals required by the body in extremely small amounts. They are: iron, iodine, copper, manganese, zinc, cobalt, molybdenum, selenium, chromium, vanadium, fluorine and silicon.

Trans fatty acids – Types of fat that are converted from their natural form into an artificial form in foods such as margines, biscuits and cakes where edible oils have been industrially hardened to ensure they stay solid at room temperature. Research suggests a strong link between trans fats and heart disease and also cancer.

TVP – Texturised vegetable protein. A type of soya product, suitable for making into mince and burgers.

Unsaturated fat – The most important fat to include in our diet. Unsaturated fats are liquid at room temperature and are divided into two groups: monounsaturated fat and polyunsaturated fat. The principal sources of monounsaturated fat are olive oil, rapeseed oil, and foods such as avocados and some nuts and seeds. Polyunsaturated fats are the vital fats. Foods high in polyunsaturates include most vegetable oils, fish oils and oily fish, nuts and seeds and their oils. The poly-unsaturates are divided further into two groups of essential fatty acids. The reason the polyunsaturated fats are so important is that the body can only receive these fatty acids through diet. This is why they are called essential. The two types of essential fatty acids (EFAs) are omega-6 and omega-3. Good sources of omega-6 are olive oil, sunflower oil, evening primrose oil, borage oil and blackcurrant oil. Good sources of omega-3 are soya bean and rapeseed oil, walnuts and walnut oil, oily fish such as salmon, mackerel, herring and fresh tuna. Essential fatty acids are vital for immune health and brain development.

Vegan – A diet that excludes all meat, fish and dairy products as well as any food derived from a living animal such as eggs. Their diet relies on beans, lentils, nuts, seeds and soya products for protein, grains and starchy vegetables for carbohydrate and nuts and seeds and oils for fat.

Vegetarian – There are two types of vegetarianism: lacto-ovo vegetarians who exclude red meat, poultry and fish and lacto-vegetarians who exclude red meat, poultry, fish and eggs.

Virus – Infectious micro-organisms that are the cause of many diseases such as the common cold, chicken pox, flu, herpes, Aids and polio. They can reproduce only by invading another living cell. A healthy cell will produce a substance called interferon which prevents the virus from spreading but in those with a weakened immune system this may not work effectively.

Resources

I have made every effort to put together a thoroughly comprehensive resources list, so that you can obtain all the ingredients and other recommendations in this book through shops, mail order or the Internet. If you have any trouble finding things you can always e-mail me via my website, www.lucyburney.com

Formula milks

Babynat organic milk: Organico, 60–62 Kings Road, Reading RG1 3AA (tel. 0118 951 0518 or visit website at www.organico.co.uk) or in all good healthfood shops.

Nanny Goat Formula, Vitacare Ltd, Unit 7, Chalcot Road, Primrose Hill, London NW1 8LH (tel. 0800 328 5826).

Organic food suppliers

Baby Organix baby foods: available nationally through supermarkets and healthfood shops. Ring 0800 393511 for a list of stockists.

Clearspring Ltd, 19A Acton Park Estate, London W3 7QE (tel. 020 8746 0152 or visit website at www.clearspring.co.uk). Mail order suppliers of Rice Dream, malt syrups, soy sauces, sweet brown rice, seaweeds, buckwheat noodles and other grocery sundries.

Graig Farm Organics, Dolau, Llandrindod Wells, Powys LD1 5TL (tel. 01597 851655 or visit website at www.graigfarm.co.uk).

Nationwide mail order for wide range of meat, game, fish and groceries.

Marigold Swiss vegetable bouillon powder: available at good supermarkets and healthfood shops, in original, low-salt and vegan versions. Distributed by Marigold Health Foods Ltd, 102 Camley Street, London NW1 0PF (tel. 020 7388 4515).

Organics Direct: Nationwide home delivery service (tel. 0845 1000 444 or order online from www.organicsdirect.co.uk). Organic fruit, vegetables and grocery suppliers (such as herb salt Herbamore by Vogel).

Oriental food suppliers: for yellow curry paste and rice paper. Look in local yellow pages for your nearest, or search the Internet for oriental supermarkets close to you.

Raw honey and tea tree (manuka) honey: from New Zealand Natural Food Co., available from healthfood shops or at Nutri Centre, 7 Park Crescent, London W1B 1PF by mail order (tel. 020 7436 5122).

Soil Association, 40–56 Victoria Street, Bristol BS1 6B7 (tel. 0117 929 0661 or visit website at www.soilassociation.org). They produce a national directory of local fruit and vegetable box schemes and home delivery.

Soya milks and yoghurts: from Provamel, available at good health-food shops and some supermarkets. Junior Yofu is a new line of calcium-enriched yoghurts suitable for babies from nine months.

Stamp Collection Foods (tel. 020 7637 5505 or visit website at www.stampcollection.co.uk). Mail order gluten-free and dairy-free products. Gluten-free flours and breads available at major super-markets. Ring for stockists.

Swaddles Green Farm, Freepost, Chard, Somerset TA20 3ZB (tel. 0845 456 1768 or visit website at www.swaddles.co.uk). Nationwide mail order organic meat, game and groceries, as well as ready meals and children's food. They have an excellent range of organic lunch box and picnic items.

Village Bakery, Melmerby, Penrith, Cumbria CA10 1HE (tel. 01768 881515 or visit website at www.village-bakery.com). Suppliers of organic breads, pastries, pies, puddings, jams and baking supplies, including plenty of wheat-free and gluten-free products via mail order or stockists throughout UK.

Vitaquell and Vitaquell Cuisine, unhydrogenated margarines available at good healthfood shops. Distributed by Brewhurst Health Food Supplies Ltd, Abbot Close, Oyster Lane, Byfleet, Surrey KT14 7SP (tel. 01932 354211).

Food supplements and herbal suppliers

BioCare: Lakeside, 180 Lifford Lane, Kings Norton, Birmingham B31 3NT (tel: 0121 433 3727). Excellent range of vitamins and minerals for breast-feeding mothers, babies and children, including Bifidobacterium Infantis (probiotic for bottle-fed babies), Strawberry Acidophilus, Vitaforte multi-vitamin and mineral powder, Dricelle flaxseed oil and fish oils, liquid vitamin and mineral drops.

East West Herb Shop: 3 Neal's Yard, Covent Garden, London WC2H 9DP (tel. 0800 092 8828). Suppliers of Gaia's Children herbal remedies for babies and children including echinacea and goldenseal formula, tummy tonic, throat spray etc., and booklet *A Parent's Guide to Children's Herbal Care* which contains ingredients, explanations and guidelines for when to use the remedies.

Enzyme Process: 4 Broadgate House, Westlode Street, Spalding PE11 2AF (tel. 01775 761927, e-mail enzymepro@compuserve.com). Suppliers of Muc Liquescence and VIR homeopathic drops.

Higher Nature: The Nutrition Centre, Burwash Common, East Sussex TN19 7LX (tel: 01435 884 668). Mail order for children's chewable multi-vitamins, Essential Balance oil and flaxseed oil (must be kept in the fridge to prevent rancidity) and Sambucol for Kids (elderberry extract).

Nutri Centre: 7 Park Crescent, London W1B 1PF (tel. 020 7436 5122 or order online from www.nutricentre.com). Mail order for full range of supplements including Biocare, Higher Nature, Solgar, Lambert's and Enzyme Process, herbs, homeopathic medicines, aromatherapy oils and flower remedies.

Revital Health shop: mail order supplier (tel. 0800 252 875) of Biosun hopi ear candles.

Verde: Mail order aromatherapy (tel. 0870 603 9186; mail order international: tel. 020 7720 1100 or visit website at www.verde.co.uk). Great aromatherapy products for babies and children including a children's chest rub, Magic Myrtle oil blend, baby soothing massage oil, Bizzy Kids bathtime soother, anti-lice sprays and oil treatment blends.

Equipment

Aquathin UK: Pure H2O Company Ltd, Unit 5, Egham Business Village, Crabtree Road, Egham, Surrey TW20 8RB (tel. 01784 221188). Suppliers and fitters of reverse osmosis water purifiers.

Brita Water Filters: jug filters available from super-markets and department stores.

Champion Juicer: imported from USA, £325 from Organics Direct (see above). Other juicers are available from department stores.

Fresh Water Company: nationwide supplier and fitter of plumbed-in water filters (tel. 020 8597 3223).

Organisations

British Allergy Foundation: Deepdene House, 30 Bellegrove Road, Welling, Kent DA16 3PY (tel. 020 8303 8525 [helpline]).

British Society of Allergy and Environmental Medicine: PO Box 7, Knighton, Powys LD7 1WT (tel. 01547 550380). Produce a list of doctors who practise nutritional and environmental medicine.

Faculty of Homeopathy: 15 Clerkenwell Close, London EC1R 0AA (tel. 020 7566 7800). Produce a list of homeopathic doctors.

The Informed Parent: PO Box 870, Harrow HA3 7UW (tel. 020 8861 1022 or visit website at www.informedparent.co.uk) Newsletter, group meetings, videos and books available regarding the pros and cons of vaccination.

Institute for Optimum Nutrition: Blades Court, Deodar Road, Putney, London SW15 2NU (tel. 020 8877 9993). Produce a list of nutrition consultants trained at the Institute.

Society of Homeopaths: 4a Artizan Road, Northampton NN1 4HU. Send an SAE for register of professional homeopaths.

Recommended Reading

Burney, Lucy, *Optimum Nutrition for Babies and Young Children*, Piatkus, 1999

Chaitow, Leon, *Vaccinations and Immunisation (What Every Parent Should Know)*, C.W. Daniel Co. Ltd, 1987 (reprinted 1994)

Charlish, Anne, *Vaccination and Immunization – What Does Your Child Need?*, Thorsons, 1996

Cochrane, Amanda, *Safe Natural Remedies for Babies and Children*, Thorsons, 1997

Cousins, Barbara, *Cooking Without*, Thorsons, 2000

Holford, Patrick, *The Optimum Nutrition Bible*, Piatkus, 1997

Immunisation against Infectious Disease, HMSO, available through mail order tel. 0870 6005522

Kenton, Leslie, *Juice High*, Ebury Press, 1996

Mendelsohn, Robert, *How to Raise a Healthy Child in Spite of Your Doctor*, Ballantine Books, 1984

Sand, Walton and Rountree, *Smart Medicine for a Healthier Child*, published by Avery and available through mail order from Nutri Centre (see above) or online from www.amazon.co.uk

Schneiber, Vera, PhD, *Vaccination: The Medical Assault on the Immune System*, 1993, available from The Informed Parent (see above)

Van Stratten, Michael, *Superjuice*, Mitchell Beazley, 1999

The WDDTY Vaccination Bible, Wallace Press; order from WDDTY (What Doctors Don't Tell You), 2 Salisbury Road, London SW19 4EZ (tel. 020 8944 9555 or online at www.wddty@zoo.co.uk)

Index